The
healing
power
of trees

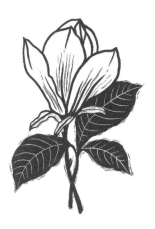

Dedication

We dedicate this book to our dear family member Mikhail Pokrepa, who unexpectedly passed around the time we started writing this book. You will always be in our hearts, reminding us that despite all the challenges we might face, we have each other to lean on, and together we can overcome any difficulties. May the bright memory of your thoughtful, compassionate nature illuminate our paths and remind us always to be kind and caring to each other.

The healing power of trees

The definitive guide to forest bathing

OLGA TEREBENINA & **GARY EVANS**

Photography by Dominick Tyler | Illustrations by Rosanna Morris

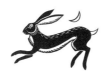

Leaping Hare Press

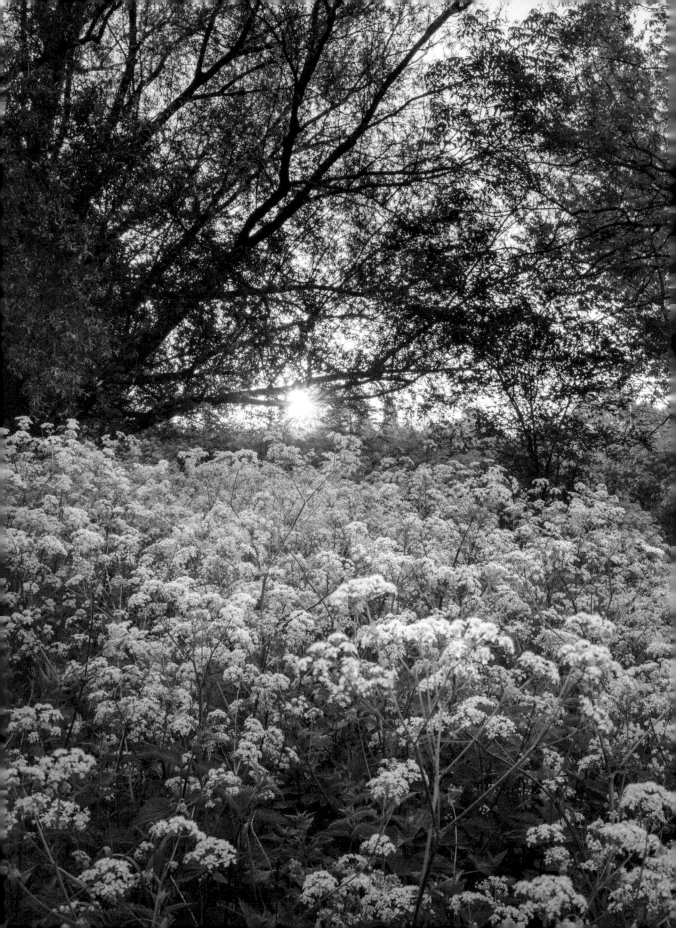

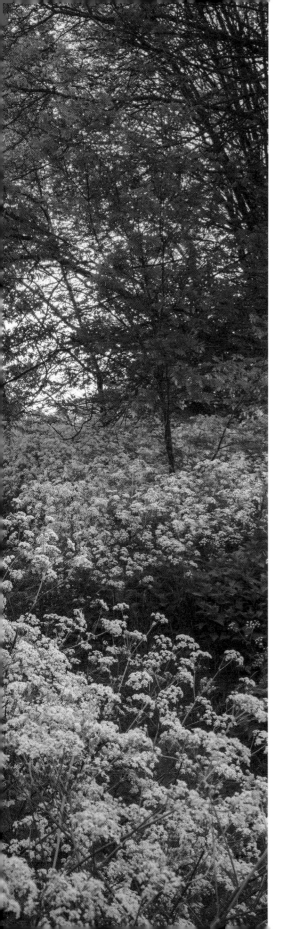

Contents

Preface

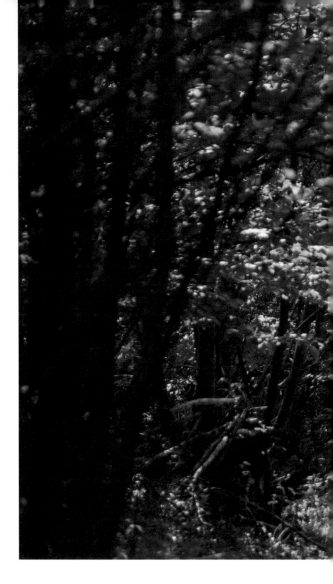

Imagine a type of practice that can boost your health and wellbeing, is widely available, has no known negative side-effects and, furthermore, can help save our planet.

Forest bathing, or *Shinrin-yoku*, is mindful time spent under the canopies of trees to benefit health and wellbeing. Its origins can be traced back to the 1980s, when the Japanese government started looking into the health and wellbeing benefits of spending time in nature as a response to an alarming stress epidemic among city workers.

From its origins in Japan, forest bathing has now spread across the globe. Some countries, such as South Korea and, increasingly, the UK, have even gone so far as to introduce it into their public welfare policies and health systems.

The benefits of forest bathing are truly spectacular – not only does it help you unwind and reduce stress, it also improves your mood and promotes better sleep. In addition, groundbreaking research has shown that forests are able to boost our immune system and even affect our physiology after only a couple of hours spent mindfully among the trees.

But how, exactly, does it work? Can anybody access these benefits? And can forest bathing really be so different from just taking a simple walk in the woods? We're here to tell you that, yes, it is different. But it is not hard to learn how to do it, and anyone can try.

Here you will find easy exercises that you can adapt for all ages, walks of life and abilities, no matter whether you live in a city or the countryside, and have hours or only a few minutes a day to spend in nature. After reading this book, you will be able to build your own robust daily forest-bathing routine and start to see how this holistic practice could change not only how you feel, but also the way you look at the outside world, including the people around you, nature and your place on this planet.

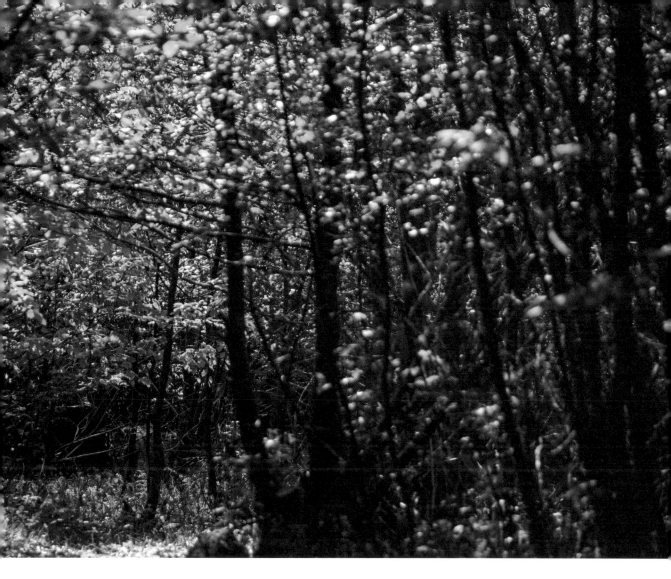

On this journey, you will be guided by world-leading forest-bathing experts who have not only experienced first hand the transformational effects of this practice on their lives, but who have also conducted groundbreaking research into the health and wellbeing benefits of a forest bathing practice, as well as witnessed its impact on the lives of thousands of people.

Alongside practical exercises and step-by-step guides, we will be sharing with you some of the reasons why forest bathing is such an effective practice, and will explain how our physiology has evolved to thrive in nature.

We will also share with you some of our stories, showing how our lives have been changed thanks to connecting with nature, and explore the impact this connection can have on our societies and the planet as a whole.

We are thrilled to have you on this journey with us and humbled to be sharing with you the magical world of forest bathing!

Olga and Gary
*Co-founders of The Forest Bathing Institute
(TFBI)*

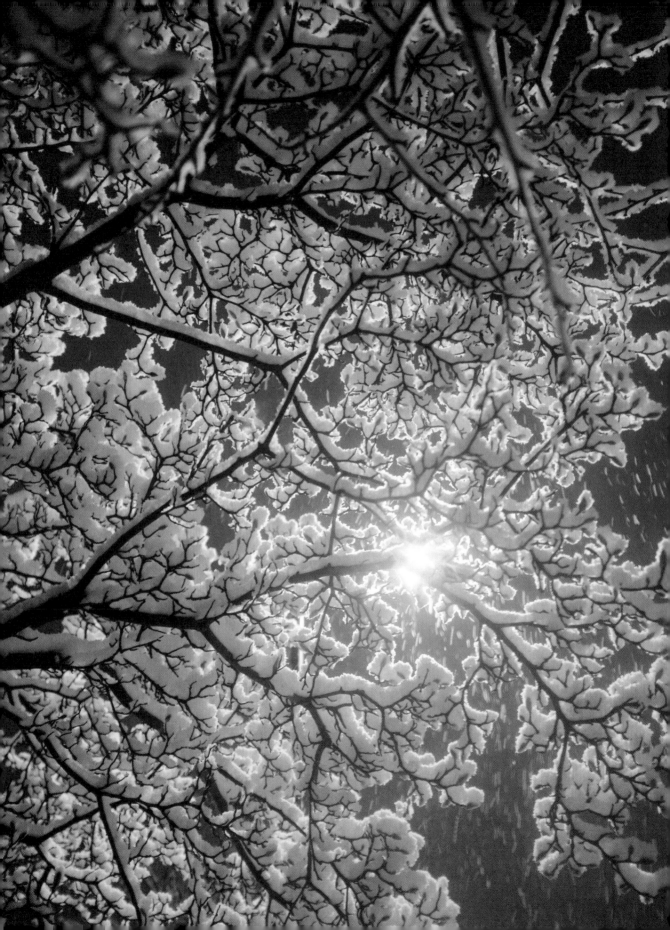

Introduction

When Olga was living in central London in 2014, she loved the vibe of the dynamic, diverse city. She was preparing for a career in the PR industry and really looking forward to working in an office in the city. Yet, slowly, day by day, nature and its gentle yet profound influence started taking root in her. And as nature was healing her on a physical and emotional level, it also started fundamentally changing who she was, her beliefs and even her dreams, just one local garden visit at a time.

I take my first step in the woods after a busy day working at my computer. The moment I enter the forest, my body instantly relaxes. My feet slow down, as if they have grown heavy, my breathing becomes deeper and slower. My senses sharpen, and it feels like I am entering a new world, a place I have never been before …

I become acutely aware of the sound of a mouse rustling in the dry grass, a distant call of a pheasant, the crisp autumn breeze on my skin … My eyes catch every pop of colour on my path, drawing my attention in. Sometimes I stop to explore, gently touching a ripening holly berry. Other times my attention is caught by the enchanting aroma of damp soil and decaying leaves, or by movement in the brambles. I wonder whether I might catch a glimpse of a deer retreating into the depth of the forest for the night.

This is the same forest I have been to many times before, yet each time I visit, it feels like I am entering a different world. Every day, the forest changes in a beautiful, never-ending dance of growth and decay. But I also change. The way I see the forest evolves each time I enter it, allowing me to see more of that magical world hidden behind the veil of the everyday hustle of life.

My forest bathing and nature connection journey began when I met Gary in 2014. At the time, I was living in central London and studying at university. And while I was academically successful and had a busy social and cultural life, I was suffering from anxiety and depression. Living in a busy city environment, combined with academic pressure and having to learn new ways of life as an immigrant in an unfamiliar city, were a lot for my body and mind to take. When Gary started showing me some of the nature connection and forest bathing techniques that helped him, I was astounded by the big difference nature made to how I felt. It was as if all the worries and noise in my head finally stopped, and I could really appreciate the beauty of nature around me.

We started by regularly visiting my local communal garden – a small green space just a couple of hundred metres away from my flat, with only a few trees. We would often simply sit on a mat on the grass underneath the trees, observing nature around us, noticing cheeky birds checking out our bags for any food scraps, feeling the sun on our skin and touching the soft grass underneath our hands.

The more I visited my local garden, the more hooked I became. Gary and I both looked forward to our daily nature outings and planned nature gateways in the glorious British countryside.

Little did I know at the time that a few years into the future, Gary and I would be newlyweds spending our honeymoon in beautiful forests in the South of France, exploring magical ancient woodlands and planning how we would set up The Forest Bathing Institute.

If you told me back in 2014 that I would be a co-founder of one of the world-leading organizations in research, education and events in forest bathing, I would not have believed you. For, indeed, my life back then was so different from what it is today and where I am now, writing this book surrounded by miles and miles of beautiful nature in the breathtaking countryside of West Sussex in the UK, on the very edge of the South Downs National Park.

I am not able to pinpoint the pivotal moment in time when I realized I no longer wanted to live in the centre of a busy city or work in a London office, but instead wanted to head an organization specializing in teaching people to connect with nature. That seed took root deep in my soul and, before I knew it, sprouted into a majestic tree that brought an abundant harvest of health and wellbeing, not only to me but also to the thousands of people whom we have helped through our work at The Forest Bathing Institute.

Nature does, indeed, work in mysterious ways! I advise you to try connecting with nature yourself, and I promise you that it will not disappoint.

Every day, the forest changes in a beautiful, never-ending dance of growth and decay. But I also change

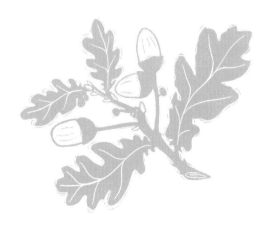

What is forest bathing?

Forest bathing, or *Shinrin-yoku*, can be described as mindful time spent under trees to promote physical and psychological health and wellbeing.

Unlike a usual walk in a forest, the pace of a forest bathing walk is much slower. Rather than aiming to be somewhere, we take time to slow down and notice things around us. There is nowhere particular to go, nowhere to be. We let our senses guide our experience of the forest, and observe what we notice with curiosity and an open mind.

This type of observation, also called mindful awareness, is one of the key components in forest bathing and is one of the main differences between a usual walk in the woods and the practice of forest bathing. It allows us to see the world around us in a different light, often highlighting things we would normally dismiss.

Interestingly, this type of mindful observation can also transcend the practice of forest bathing and spill into our wider lives, allowing us to see ourselves, as well as the people and circumstances around us, in a different light. This makes it a truly holistic practice that brings about wellbeing.

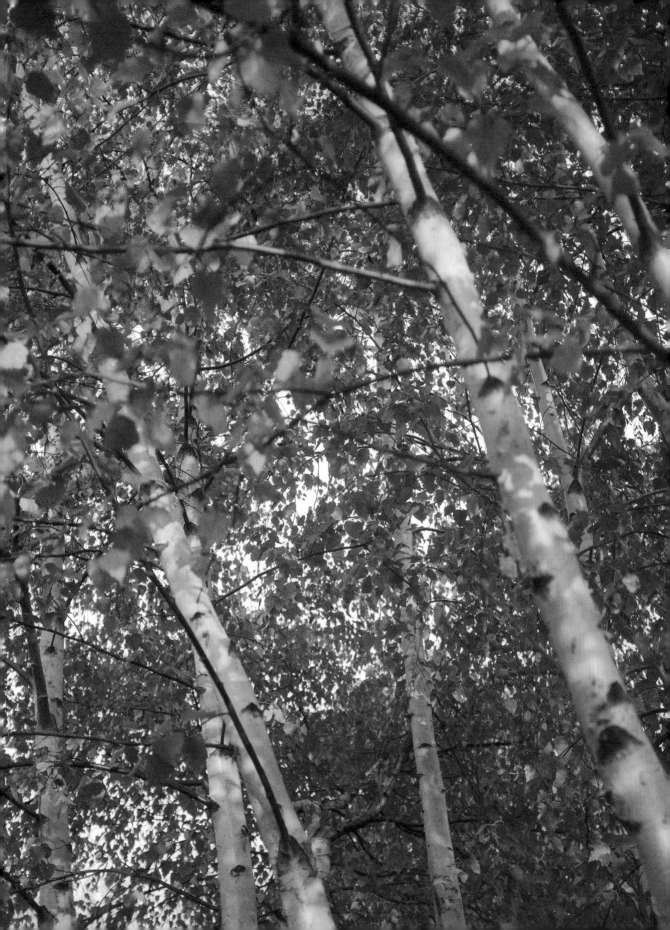

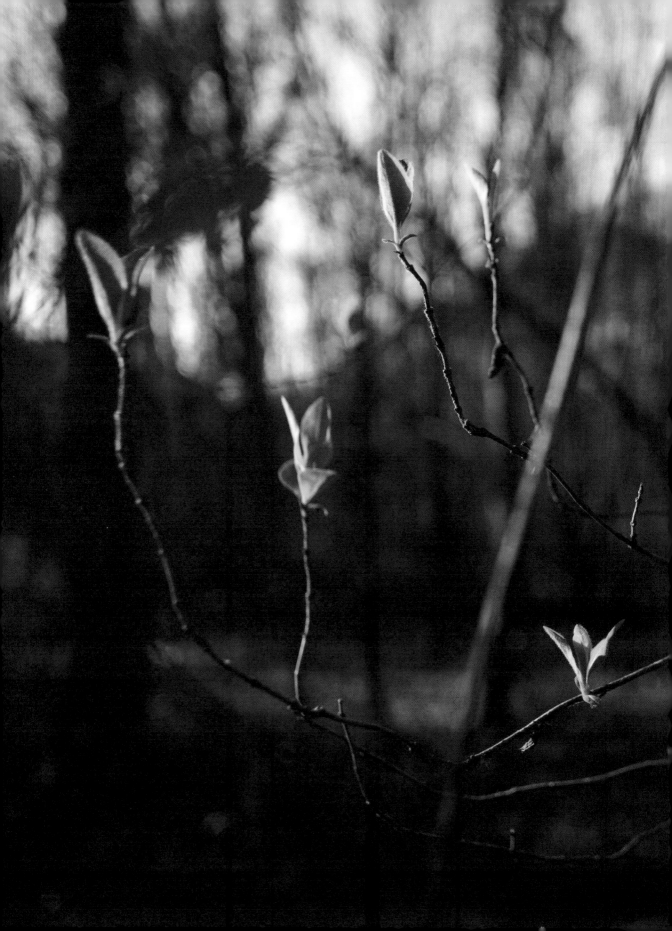

Origins

The term *Shinrin-yoku* (*shinrin*: forest; *yoku*: bath or bathing) was coined in 1982 by Tomohide Akiyama, who, at the time, was the Director of the Japanese Ministry of Agriculture, Forestry and Fisheries. In the 1980s and 1990s, while Japan was experiencing rapid economic growth, it also saw an epidemic of stress due to long working hours and high-performance demands from employers.

The Japanese government started researching solutions to the stress epidemic and, as around 70 per cent of Japan is covered in forests and trees, it was only natural that the government's attention was caught by the potential of nature, and specifically forests, to help reduce stress and boost health and wellbeing.

When Japan first introduced forest bathing, little research was done into its benefits. So, in 2004, the Japanese government asked Professor Qing Li, based at the Nippon Medical School in Tokyo, to research the health benefits of forest bathing. The following year he conducted the first forest bathing study in Japan, in Iiyama City.[1] Since then, Professor Li has become a leading figure in Japanese research into *Shinrin-yoku*. He has published countless research papers that evidence the physiological and mental health benefits of spending time in a forest, from which a new branch of medicine – forest medicine, which includes *Shinrin-yoku* – has emerged. Further research has been conducted globally, including by The Forest Bathing Institute in cooperation with some of the UK's leading universities.

Professor Li is an inspiration for us here at The Forest Bathing Institute, and in 2023 he was appointed our Scientific Advisor. In his book, *Shinrin-Yoku: The Art and Science of Forest Bathing* (see page 214), Professor Li beautifully captures the benefits and experiences of forest bathing.

Today, *Shinrin-yoku* is a well-known public health intervention in Japan, and is used by millions of people a year to treat conditions such as high blood pressure, anxiety and stress. Indeed, across Japan there are over 65 accredited Forest Therapy Trails where individuals, some of whom may have been referred for a particular health condition, can follow dedicated woodland trail routes that have been assessed for their health-giving properties.

At these sites, participants are met by medical professionals who conduct an assessment, which might involve measuring blood pressure and potentially taking a blood sample. Following the participants' two- to three-hour walk along the woodland therapy trail, their measurements are reassessed to monitor any changes that may have taken place. At this stage, they may be advised to continue their *Shinrin-yoku* programme to assist with ongoing nature therapy treatment for their condition.

From Japan, forest bathing spread to South Korea, where the government faced similar problems of stress and burnout among its workers due to unprecedented technological development, urbanization and economic growth. South Korea saw potential in forest bathing not only for city workers, but also for other members of the population, including children in schools and nurseries, and pregnant women.

Forest bathing has also started to spread to other parts of the globe, including California and elsewhere in the United States, as well as Europe. Although *Shinrin-yoku* was initially understood as a holistic wellbeing practice with the emphasis on its potential within preventive medicine, it has since gained more recognition and more interest from researchers at leading universities, health care systems and even governments. Clinical research has now started in these countries too, and this is something we at The Forest Bathing Institute are delighted to be involved with.

In the UK, forest bathing is now part of Green Social Prescribing in the county of Surrey. What this means is that if you go to your healthcare provider and they decide that forest bathing could be helpful to your condition, you can be referred to a session.

With the rise in interest in environmental protection, forest bathing has gained yet another group of followers – those who can see how, by accessing the health and wellbeing benefits of nature, we as a society will not only be able to increase savings on public healthcare but also help protect the planet. Time spent in nature invariably inspires people to want to protect it, especially if those people feel grateful as a result of feeling the wellbeing benefits shared by nature. We have a natural instinct to protect what we care about.

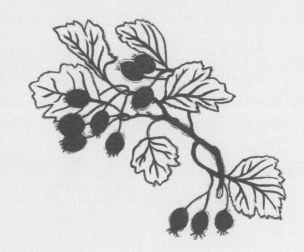

Shinrin-yoku and Shintoism

Even though *Shinrin-yoku* as a term did not exist before the 1980s, people in Japan have always had a strong relationship with nature. Shinto, one of the main religions in Japan, revolves around the notion of *kamis*, supernatural entities that are found in all things, including natural elements.

The Shinto religion emphasizes the relationship between humans and nature, land and environment, cultivating a respectful attitude towards the natural world.

In Shinto, a *shinboku*, literally translated as 'god tree', is a tree or a forest that is worshipped at, or near, a Shinto shrine (temple).

Apart from Shintoism, many indigenous cultures, including First Nations groups, possess deeply intertwined relationships with nature, imbuing it with sacredness and encouraging respect and careful stewardship. Indigenous cosmologies often emphasize the interconnectedness of all living things, viewing humans as part of a larger ecological web, rather than separate from it.

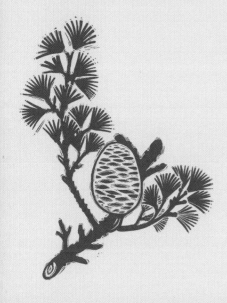

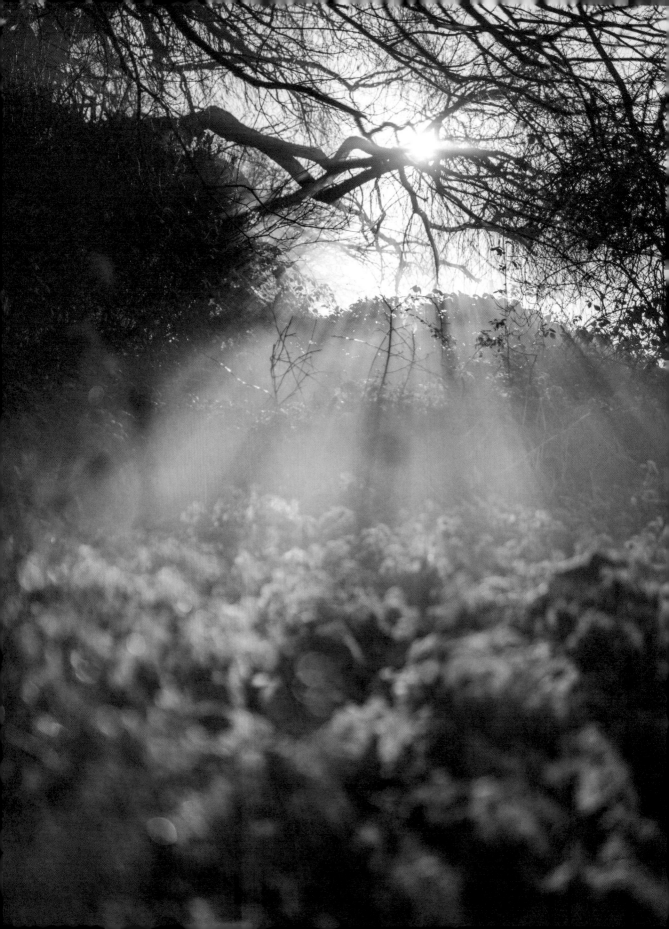

Health and
wellbeing benefits

The research on the benefits of forest bathing has only just started, with more benefits being discovered every year. So far, it's been shown forest bathing can help to:

- Reduce blood pressure
- Lower stress
- Improve cardiovascular and metabolic health
- Lower blood sugar levels
- Improve concentration and memory
- Lift depression
- Improve pain thresholds
- Improve energy
- Boost the immune system with an increase in the count of the body's natural killer (NK) cells
- Increase anti-cancer protein production
- Lose weight

The amazing thing about forest bathing is that while it has been shown to have so many potential health and wellbeing benefits, no contraindications have yet been recorded. Another incredible thing about forest bathing is how versatile it is. While it is true that the environment can play a significant role in the rewards you can get from forest bathing – for instance, time spent in an ancient woodland with a rich variety of flora and fauna might bring extra advantages – anyone can benefit from the practice. And sometimes, we can benefit from it even if we can't get into a forest – in this book, we will show you how.

Disclaimer

Please note that the forest bathing exercises provided in this book are only meant as a general introduction to forest bathing practice for you, your family and your friends. This information is for general knowledge and informational purposes only and does not constitute medical advice. The information provided in this book is not a substitute for professional medical advice, diagnosis or treatment, and is not intended to cure or prevent any disease. Always seek the advice of your doctor or other qualified healthcare provider with any questions you may have regarding a medical condition or health concerns, and before making any decisions related to your health or treatment, or starting any new diet, exercise programme or other health-related activities. Never disregard professional medical advice or delay in seeking it.

If you need clarification on the exercises or whether they suit your needs, we advise you to consult your health provider and a qualified forest bathing guide. As the exercises in this book are intended for general public use, it is not possible to take into account individual differences and needs. If you have physical or mental health concerns, please consult your healthcare provider regarding starting a forest bathing practice.

All exercises presented in this book are suggestions only. Always take care, and never exceed your limit; stop if physical or emotional discomfort arises and contact your health care provider. The exercises provided in this book are not intended as training to guide others in forest bathing; if you would like to do so, we advise you to seek a certified training course in forest bathing guiding.

Please note that individual results may vary. Any use of the information in this book is at the reader's discretion and risk. The author and publisher make no representations or warranties with respect to the accuracy, completeness or fitness for a particular purpose of the contents of this book and exclude all liability to the extent permitted by law for any errors and omissions and for any injury, loss, damage or expense suffered by anyone arising out of the use, or misuse, of the information in this book, or any failure to take professional medical advice.

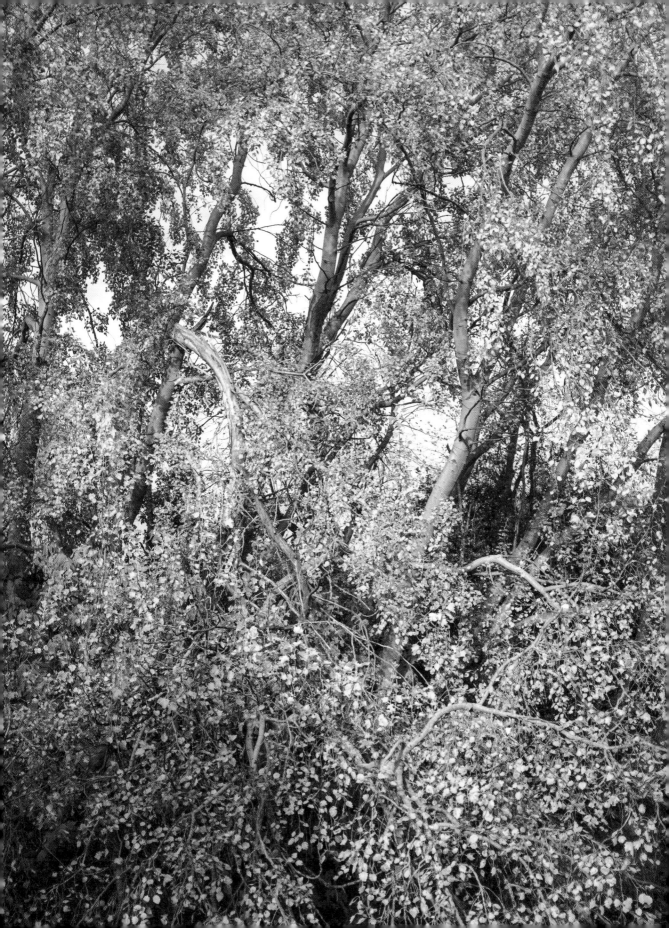

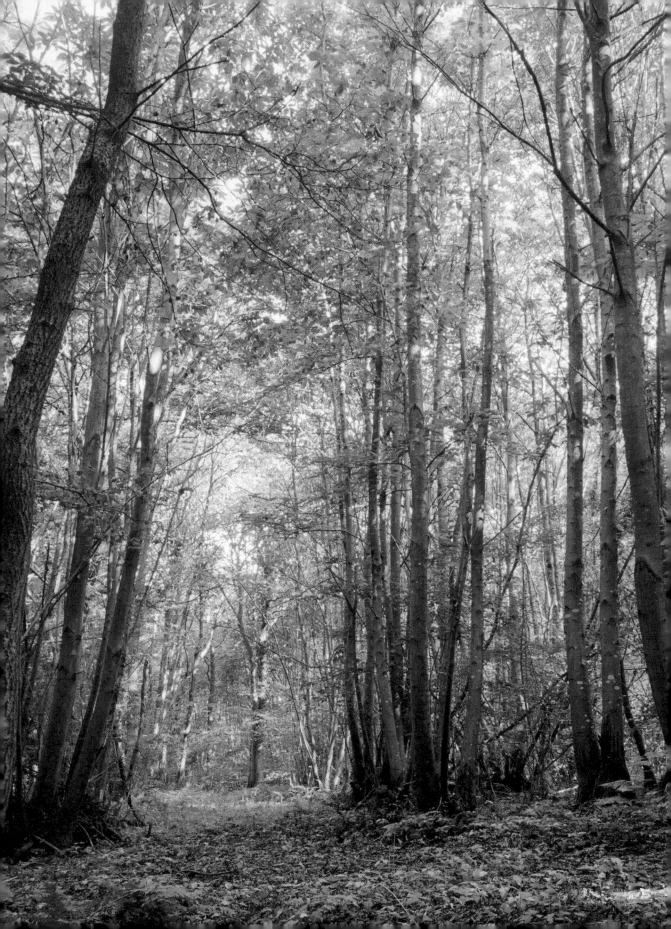

Chapter one

Why nature feels good

Before we think about how to implement forest bathing in our everyday lives, it might be helpful to understand how our physiology has (or, more importantly, has not) evolved over time.

While our physiology has changed little over the last millennium, our way of life has changed enormously. No one would deny that the technological developments of modernization have led to great discoveries and opportunities; however, the downside of progress is that our bodies often struggle to keep up with the pace.

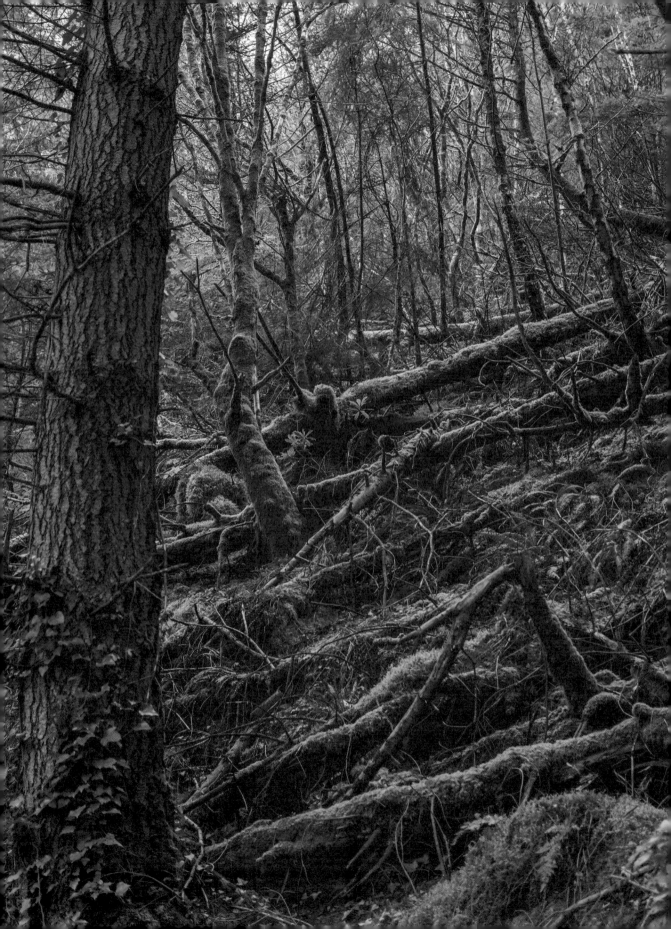

The interesting fact about humans is that our physiology has not changed much for thousands of years. Early humans lived as hunter-gatherers until approximately 12,000 years ago, when agriculture began to develop. If you consider that the Industrial Revolution, arguably the crucible for the infrastructures and cities of our modern world, only began in the late eighteenth century, you can appreciate that the vast majority of our history as a species has been spent in close proximity to nature.

As a result of this timeline, despite the rapid changes of the recent centuries brought about by modernization, technological developments and urbanization, our physiology is hardwired to function optimally in natural environments, rather than in the industrialized world.

It is no surprise, then, that the human eye can distinguish the most shades of the colour green (it has been theorized this may have been an evolutionary trait that enabled us to tell the difference between edible and poisonous plants). That we are designed to operate in natural environments also explains why some studies show a strong correlation between access to green space, self-reported wellbeing and even physical health. Researchers have found that, on average, individuals have both lower mental distress and better wellbeing when living in urban areas with more green space.[2]

Furthermore, over time human physiology seems to have evolved in such a way that natural cues (such as birdsong and running water) appear to produce a relaxing sensation in our body when we're walking in nature, while modern city cues provoke the reaction of alertness.

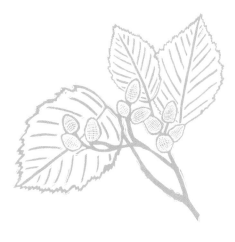

Stress grows as life speeds up

The key to understanding what is happening in our bodies when we go about our everyday lives is the autonomic nervous system. It has two main branches. One branch is responsible for rest, relaxation and homeostasis (a state of balance among all body systems, needed for the body to function correctly), and we call it the parasympathetic nervous system. The other branch is responsible for keeping us alert and aware (for example, helping us meet that last-minute deadline or even avoid a car crash) and is known as the sympathetic nervous system, or the 'fight-flight-or-freeze' branch.

Ideally, we should be spending around 80 per cent of our time in parasympathetic nervous system activity – actively relaxed, at ease, peaceful and happy. No lions to chase us, no last-minute deadlines to complete. However, with the speed of life that we are currently experiencing, the sympathetic nervous system seems to have taken over and many of us can spend 60–80 per cent of our time caught up in fight-flight-or-freeze.

If you take a moment to think about the pace of your everyday life, would you say that you find it stressful? From the moment we get up in the morning, we face more potential stressors than any generation before us. For instance, if you think about your normal morning, how would you describe it? Perhaps it is calm and peaceful, and you feel that you manage to do all your tasks in your own time? Or maybe you feel that some mornings are more of a flow, while others can be fast-paced and challenging? Or maybe every morning you can think of is a struggle – from waking up, to trying to fit in time to have a decent breakfast, to running a dozen family errands, always waiting to have a cup of tea for that much-needed break? The reality of things is, given the pace of progress and future projections, the speed at which we live is only likely to increase over time.

The Japanese government started noticing this rise in stress levels in the 1980s, when nearly 80 per cent of the population moved from villages into major cities and towns.

With the pressures from the economy, from modernization, from urbanization and technological development, more and more workers began to see their stress levels increase, leading to a concomitant increase in stress-related illnesses and even deaths.

In the modern day, recent surveys show an increase in the number of employees experiencing moderate to high stress. One report, which collected data covering all areas of wellbeing from 4,170 employees across the globe, from different demographics and a variety of employment sectors, found that the number of employees experiencing moderate to high stress increased from 67 per cent in 2022 to 76 per cent in 2023.[3]

Unfortunately, these numbers are only likely to increase in the future with the growing pressures of modern life.

The reality of things is, given the pace of progress and future projections, the speed that we live at is only likely to increase over time

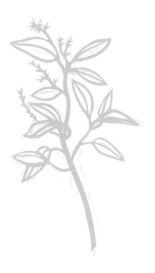

'Technostress'

In the 1980s, the Japanese government identified the use of technology, or rather the stress induced by the use (or overuse) of technology – 'technostress' – as a problem. 'Technostress' refers to the negative psychological and emotional impact that arises from the use of technology. It can manifest as feelings of anxiety, frustration and overwhelm caused by factors such as information overload, constant connectivity and difficulty adapting to new technologies. Technostress can affect individuals in both personal and professional settings.

With the growing demand to stay connected, technology has become a tool that can be all too easily overused.

Of course technology has many vital uses. Improved communications mean we are able to reach people whom we likely would never have met before. Our lives have been simplified, and we can progress further in so many areas, including science and commerce, to name just two. But it would be naive to suggest that there wasn't also a downside.

Technostress puts yet further pressure on our bodies and minds, demanding faster reactions and more optimized functioning. Phones and computers become more and more sophisticated, while our bodies receive little to no upgrade. The result of this is an epidemic of stress that we can now see worldwide.

And technology doesn't just affect our mental health. There are other ways in which it has an impact on us; for example, some of us might notice that we experience discomfort or even pain from prolonged use of technology. There's also the issue of sleep. Using technology too close to bedtime can cause sleep problems due to blue light exposure suppressing the production of melatonin, a hormone that helps regulate sleep-wake cycles. This can make it harder to fall asleep and can disrupt the quality of our slumber.

The great thing about forest bathing is that is has been shown to positively affect stress, anxiety, mood and rumination of thought. Not only that, natural light exposure can be a gentle aid to regulate circadian rhythms, increase production of melatonin and help you fall asleep at night.

Technostress is a modern malaise that is unlikely to get better – very few of us, after all, can completely get away from technology – but forest bathing has great potential to help with the stress, anxiety, sleep issues and sensory overload that can accompany it.

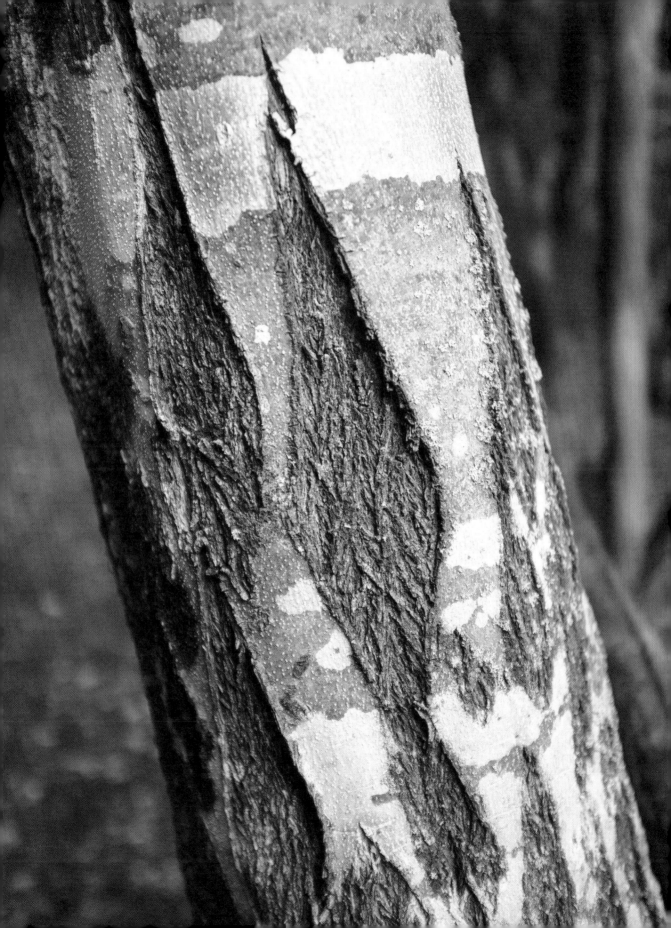

Mindfulness: the key to changing our body's reactions

While we are unable to control the speed at which the world is progressing and functioning, we can control our reactions to it. For example, we can schedule in some 'screen free' time, take breaks from social media and filter out some influences we think might be unhealthy. However, while we may be able to control our conscious reactions, our inbuilt physiological processes that are triggered by changes in the environment probably need more work, understanding and structure.

Many of us live our lives at such a fast pace that slowing down seems like a luxury we cannot afford. With burnout looming on the horizon, though, one could equally claim the opposite – that in a fast-paced world which only seems to be getting faster every day, we cannot afford not to slow down. Indeed, recent statistics show that stress is at a record high. No wonder so many people nowadays are looking for solutions to better manage stress levels. Wouldn't it be great if there was a practice that would enable us to function at our optimum and sharpen our attention, while allowing our busy minds to naturally slow down when they need to? Fortunately there is!

Mindfulness can be described as paying attention to the present moment – also known as moment-to-moment awareness – including the world around us (people, animals, nature, objects) and our bodily sensations, feelings and emotions in a nonjudgemental way.

Mindfulness is often associated with meditation, one of its more formal practices, but it can in fact have different faces. You can adopt a mindful attitude even when performing the most mundane of tasks, for example, washing dishes, gardening, jogging or working. Any activity can potentially be enhanced by doing it mindfully – not only does it allow us to slow down, but it also allows us to notice things we might have missed before, and better appreciate little everyday joys.

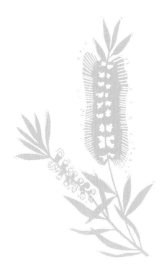

An overall review of mindfulness-based interventions has concluded that they are effective in improving many biopsychosocial conditions, including depression, anxiety, stress, insomnia, pain, weight control and prosocial behaviours, amongst others.[4]

Mindfulness is now used across different fields – from programmes targeted at helping people reduce stress, like Mindfulness Based Stress Reduction (MBSR), to teaching kids mindfulness at school as a technique to aid concentration and induce the relaxed-yet-alert state that is perfect for learning. More corporations are now also using mindfulness as a technique not only to boost their employees' performance, but also to decrease absenteeism and promote a better work environment for their employees.

Interestingly, while mindfulness can be included in virtually all aspects of our lives, when it is combined with spending time in nature, such as through forest bathing, it seems to produce extra benefits. A study we took part in, led by Associate Professor Kirsten McEwan at the University of Derby, compared the benefits of indoor mindfulness activities with forest bathing, and found that the latter produced potentially greater and more accessible results, especially for beginners.[5]

This is not to say that indoor mindfulness activities are not helpful. We are enthusiastic proponents of all types of mindfulness, as long as they are carried out correctly and practised responsibly. However, it is really exciting to know that, while time spent in nature and mindfulness each have their own separate benefits, combining the two practices seems to create additional benefits.

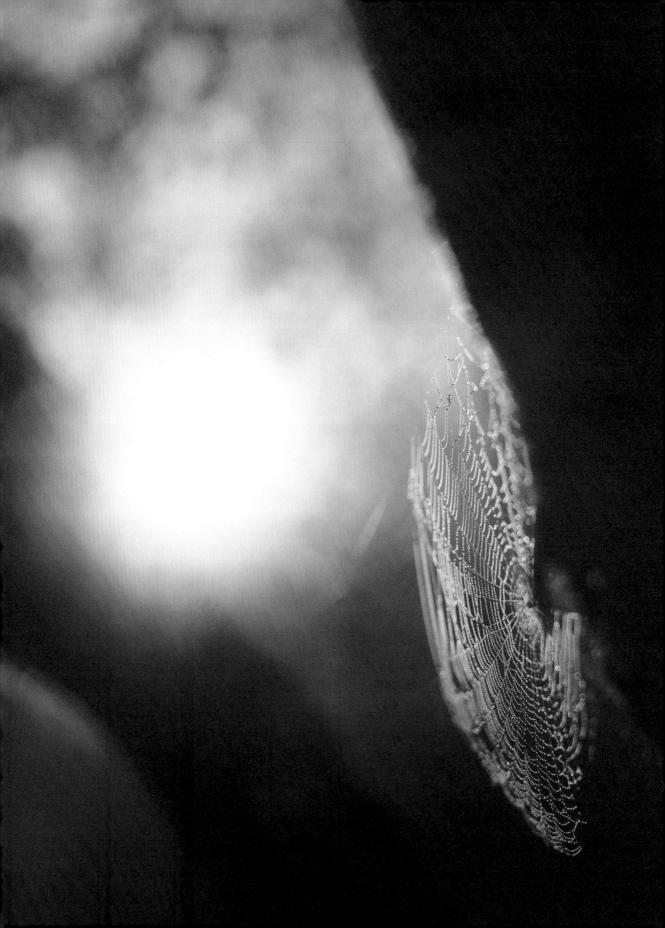

How to be mindful in a forest

The good news about mindfulness is that everyone can do it. No special training is required, although if you would like to have some it can add extra benefits. In fact, you might be surprised to hear that you could be practising mindfulness already!

Don't believe us? Well, have you have ever experienced any of the following:

- Being taken in by the beauty of the surrounding landscape?
- Stopping to listen to the sound of a bird in the distance?
- Feeling the warmth of the spring sun on your face?
- Enjoying the refreshing dew of the early morning?
- Stopping to watch a bird fly past?
- Listening to the sound of the rain?
- Watching a sunset?
- Watching animals grazing or at play?
- Planting seeds and plants and feeling empathy for the life you are nurturing?

If you ticked off one or more from the list – congratulations! You have already experienced moments of being mindful in nature. I will also go so far as to say that if in any of those moments you were in a forest, you were likely practising forest bathing! Easy, isn't it?

However, if you have not experienced any of the things on the list and, in fact, can't even remember the last time you felt the sun on your skin, do not worry. Throughout this book, we will guide you step-by-step and show you how to build and develop your nature connection and start practising forest bathing, one walk at a time.

The senses: gateway to mindfulness

There are many ways in which you can practise mindfulness, but using your senses to slow down and connect with the environment can be one of the most accessible. When forest bathing, not only will you be practising mindfulness, you will also be reaping all the amazing benefits of being outdoors. And helping to protect nature. A true win-win!

While some of us who have tried meditation indoors might have found our minds wandering (which is normal) and may even have been close to giving up altogether (or perhaps did), mindfulness in nature can be a gentler way to start a mindfulness practice, especially if you have a busy mind.

One of the reasons for this is that when we practise meditation indoors we tend to shut ourselves off from any sensory distractions. This can be a great exercise and has so many benefits, especially at the beginning stages of the practice, but the downside is that the mind can sometimes get easily distracted and start to wander. As a result, many beginners give up early, without giving mindfulness a chance.

Forest bathing, in contrast to indoor types of mindfulness practice, does not require you to shut out any distractions. On the contrary, we are often guided by these 'distractions' and make them our moment-to-moment points of anchor in our mindfulness practice.

One moment, we could be focusing on the song of a bird sitting on a branch. Another moment, we feel the change in the wind and pause to feel it caressing our skin. Then we might observe squirrels playing in the leaves, a blackbird rustling in the bushes, lush moss waiting to be explored through touch … The amazing thing about nature is that it is captivating. We have simply forgotten where, or rather *how*, to look.

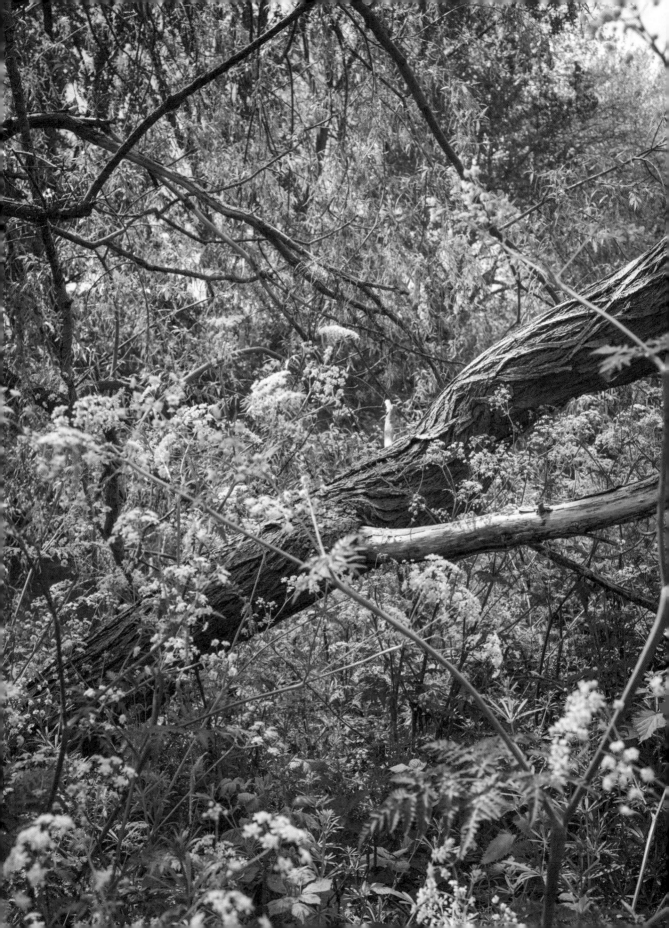

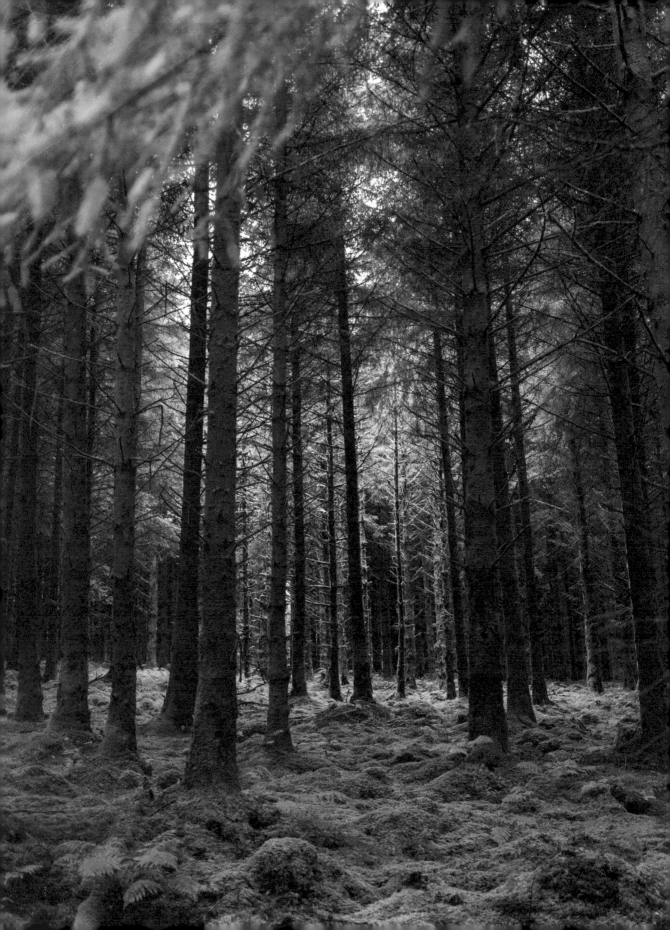

Relearning how to be in nature

At The Forest Bathing Institute, we re-educate people, teaching them what to do in nature. As kids, we know this instinctively. If you look back to your time as a child, you might remember some moments spent in nature – maybe on a family walk in a local park, helping your grandparents in their garden, swimming in the river or going on a camping trip with your school. The interesting thing is that for most of us, the memories are often very happy – moments of joy, excitement, fun and exploration, free from worry!

However, while we may have wonderful memories of these times spent in nature, we do not necessarily remember all the details of what exactly we did, or these are not the main part of our memories. Instead, it is the feelings of joy and happiness, the momentary excitement, that are often at the forefront. And if we were then asked, 'How do we replicate those moments?', many of us might answer – there is no way, it is all in the past now ...

The good news is that it is not just in the past. At The Forest Bathing Institute, we have seen first-hand from running sessions for thousands of people that creating those moments of happiness is easy – it is literally at your fingertips! And once you rediscover this ability, you will be surprised you ever forgot it. Anyone, anywhere, at any point in their lives, can learn how to do it. The only thing we ask is that you be open-minded, and allow a little bit of magic and curiosity into your life. Nature will do the rest.

The only thing we ask is that you be open-minded, and allow a little bit of magic and curiosity into your life. Nature will do the rest

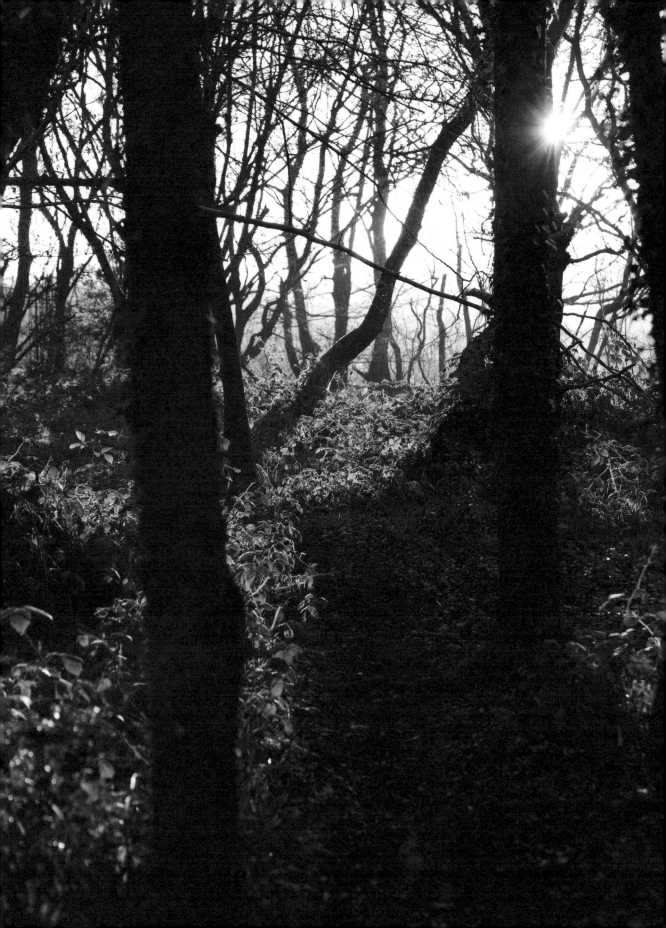

Chapter two

Starting your forest bathing practice

Now that you know about some of the benefits of forest bathing, hopefully you are keen to give it a go! But how do you do it? What do you need to bring with you? What if you don't have a forest near you? And what if it rains? In this chapter, we will be covering some of the basics to help you get started with your forest bathing practice.

The Nature Pyramid

The concept of the Nature Pyramid, first developed by Tanya Denckla Cobb at the University of Virginia, emphasizing different levels of engagement with nature for overall wellbeing, is a modern framework inspired by various disciplines including psychology, environmental education and ecopsychology. It builds upon the growing body of research and practices highlighting the numerable benefits of nature experiences for human health and happiness.

While the Nature Pyramid does not have a single definite origin, it is influenced by the broader movement promoting nature-based interventions, ecotherapy and nature-connectedness practices aimed at enhancing human wellbeing and environmental conservation. The pyramid serves as a practical guide for individuals seeking to cultivate a more meaningful relationship with nature and to integrate its healing qualities into their lives.

Similar to the food pyramid that illustrates the importance of a balanced diet, the Nature Pyramid highlights different levels of nature experiences that individuals can incorporate into their lives for optimal health and happiness. These range from daily interactions to less frequent but more immersive wilderness experiences. By engaging with nature regularly and in diverse ways, individuals can reap the physical, mental and emotional benefits of spending time outdoors and fostering a deeper connection with the natural world.

On the opposite page we share with you a general outline of what the Nature Pyramid could look like, as based on Dr Rachel Hopman's 20-5-3 rule highlighted in Michael Easter's book.[6]

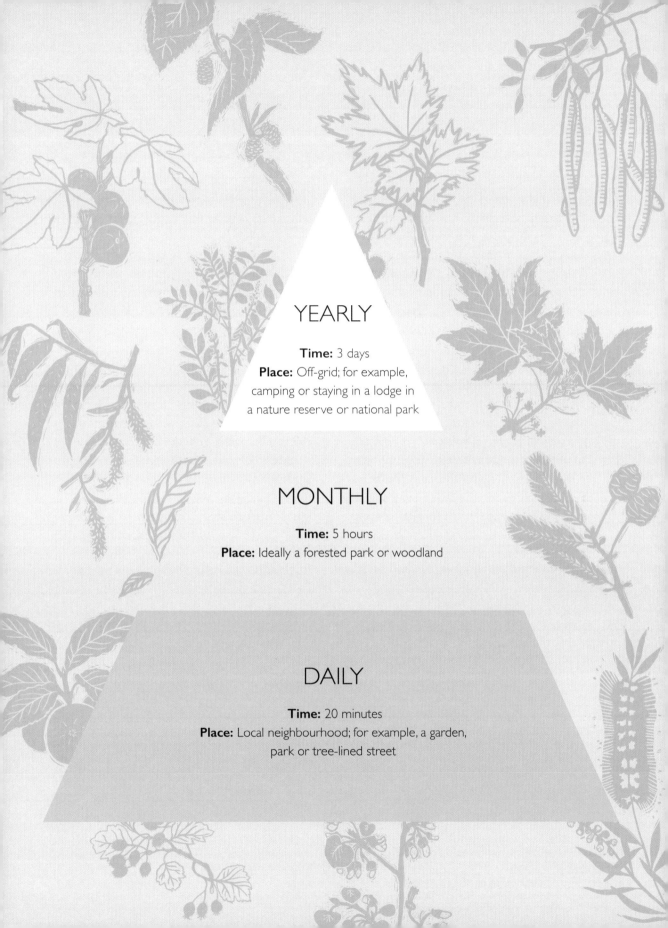

YEARLY

Time: 3 days
Place: Off-grid; for example,
camping or staying in a lodge in
a nature reserve or national park

MONTHLY

Time: 5 hours
Place: Ideally a forested park or woodland

DAILY

Time: 20 minutes
Place: Local neighbourhood; for example, a garden,
park or tree-lined street

Twenty minutes daily

The good news is you do not necessarily need to change your current lifestyle much to start seeing benefits from spending time in nature.

The research shows that as little as 20 minutes of nature immersion a day can bring about favourable changes. A recent study by Dr Hopman concluded that just a 20-minute walk through a city botanical garden can enhance cognition and memory, and improve general feelings of wellbeing. (She also noted, however, that people who use their mobile phones during the walk did not experience the benefits.[7]) These findings were reaffirmed by a study at the University of Michigan, showing that as little as 20 minutes in nature three times a week resulted in an efficient decrease in stress hormones. The optimal time was found to be between 20 and 30 minutes, and benefits continued to accrue after 30 minutes, though at a reduced rate.[8]

The miraculous benefits of just 20 minutes in nature are explained by the 'soft fascination' mode that our brain enters when in nature. This mode is associated with resetting our brain after periods of intense focus, which helps us think, process information and problem-solve more effectively.

The great thing about this finding is that you do not necessarily need to go into a forest to reap the benefits of forest bathing; you don't even need to visit a park! A simple stroll down a tree-lined street can be enough to kick-start the 'soft fascination' mode. Just make sure you put your phone away, as even notifications can switch your brain out of the 'soft fascination' mode.

You can discover more details on how you can dedicate 20 minutes daily to a forest bathing practice in the 'Find the time' section on page 188.

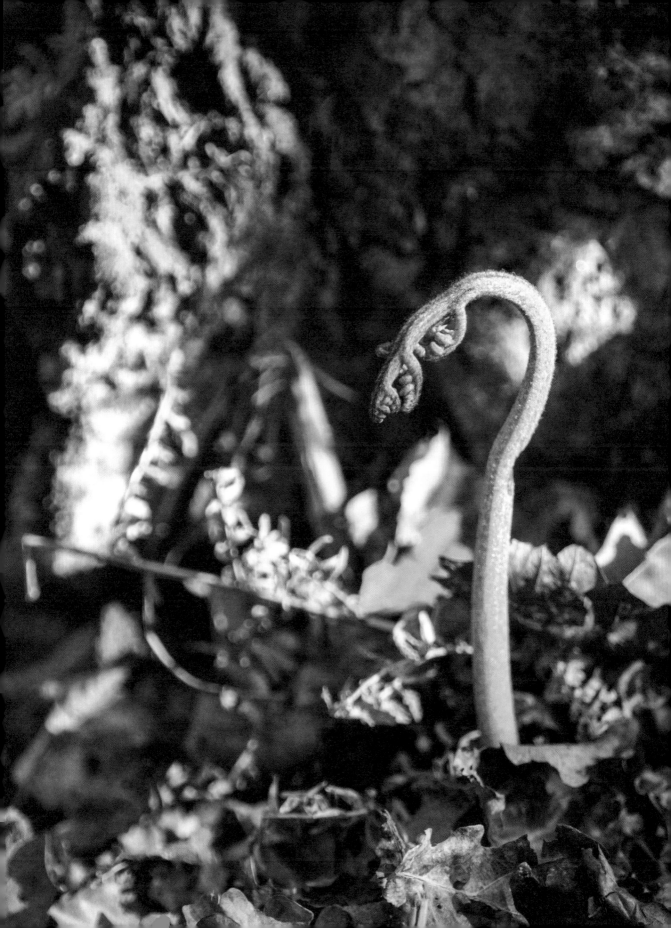

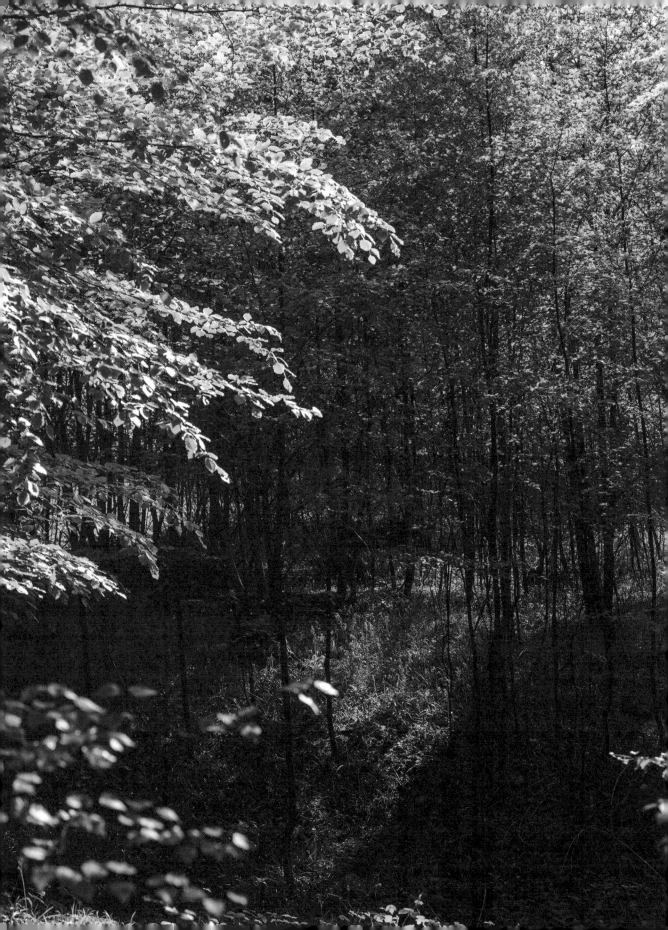

Five hours each month

A 2005 survey in Finland concluded that city dwellers felt less stressed and happier when they had at least five hours of nature exposure a month – and that a greater amount of exposure brought extra benefits.[9]

Another study conducted by the Finnish government in 2014 compared how people felt in three different environments: a city centre, a city park and a forested park.[10] The conclusion was that people who spent time in a city park felt more relaxed than the people in a city centre, and those who went to a forested park felt the most relaxed out of the three groups.

According to Hopman, the reason for this is a combination of many things. City environments are normally associated with louder sounds (think of the sound of a siren), a faster pace and sharp angles, while natural environments tend to be quieter and slower paced and instead of sharp angles, offer us fractal patterns, which our brain finds especially relaxing.

While the environment might play a big role in the quality of the benefits we get from nature exposure (the more natural or wilder it is, the better), many other factors are important. For instance, while it is ideal if you can find an ancient or semi-ancient woodland that you can visit at least once a month, this might not always be practical. If getting to this woodland involves too much energy or the commute there is too expensive and/or stressful, or if you simply are not enjoying that location, you might benefit more in an environment that is less wild but which you can easily access. It is all about the balance.

We will talk more about the different environments where you can practise forest bathing in the next chapters.

Three days every year

Three days is the ideal amount of time we should be spending outdoors off-grid every year. This could be camping or renting a cabin in a nature reserve or national park, on your own or with family and friends.

In his research, Professor Li has found out that the immune system experiences a dramatic boost, demonstrated by an increased NK (natural killer) cell activity, after three days and two nights of forest immersion.[11] This increased cell activity lasted for more than one month after the immersion (suggesting that one trip every month would be the ideal schedule to maintain a consistently higher level of NK activity).

When we spend a few days in a forested environment, coupled with the effects of abstaining from technology, we are likely to experience benefits to our health and wellbeing, including improved sleep, reduced stress, clearer thinking and even an improved ability to focus and think creatively.

Spending three days immersed in nature will look different for each of us. For some, it could be as simple as camping out in our back garden. However, if you are able to go a bit further with this, you can try camping out in a dedicated camping site, or opt for lodges, preferably situated in a wooded area or a national park.

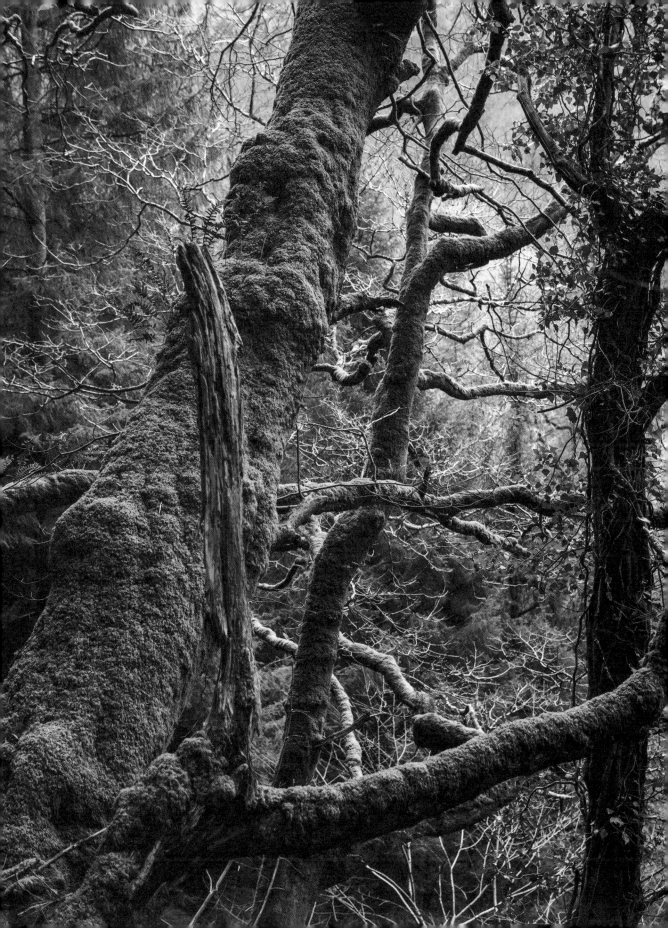

Principles of forest bathing

There are no concrete rules for practising forest bathing, and we always say that no one session is the same as another. This is because the weather, our individual differences, how we feel, and what we think or like changes from day to day, and sometimes even from hour to hour! For instance, if you have a challenging conversation with your partner and then try to go to nature to help you calm down, you might find it takes you longer to tune in to the environment than it might have done the day before, when you hadn't experienced any significant events beforehand.

However, our day-to-day circumstances ebb and flow, and we can still benefit from spending time in nature. In the following pages, we share some tips aimed to help you with this.

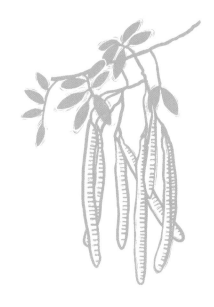

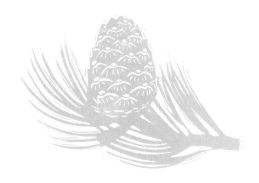

Stay silent

While you might want to take someone with you when going for a walk (advisable if you are going somewhere you don't know that well), we suggest you stay silent for the duration of the forest bathing practice. Sharing the experience with another person can be a big part of forest bathing and has been shown to have many great benefits, in particular helping our body swap to parasympathetic nervous system activity, which encourages rest and relaxation. One of the findings in our 2019 study with the University of Derby was that HRV (heart rate variability) readings were highest (indicating less stress, see page 111) during three activities, one of which was sharing in a group (the other two were listening to the sound of running water and hugging a tree).[12] However, while you are in the process of observing and connecting with nature, it really is best to stay as silent as you can. As well as providing an opportunity to hear the natural sounds around you, silence is a great facilitator of slowing the mind.

Keeping silent throughout the forest bathing walk can help you become more engaged with the environment, allowing you to tune in to what is happening around you. You are more likely to notice a beautiful flower or spot a deer in the distance. When our focus is on nature, it allows us to engage more and on a deeper level with our surroundings, which can potentially bring greater benefits and joy to the practice.

For safety reasons we would recommend bringing a phone with you whenever you are out, so that you are covered in case of emergency. However, while you are practising forest bathing, even if it is for just 15 minutes, we recommend switching your phone to silent if you can, to avoid distractions.

Slow down

Many of us might be used to a brisk pace – for instance, when walking our dog, jogging or hurrying to be somewhere at a certain time – but forest bathing refers to a leisurely walk in nature.

What this means is that, for many of us, we will need to slow down the pace of our walk quite a bit. At the beginning, some might find this a bit uncomfortable, even frustrating. However, with practice, as you gradually slow down, you might find that you are enjoying this new, slower pace, and the upside is that you might be able to notice more things around you as you walk.

Walking slowly has a few benefits. Firstly, as mentioned before, it can allow us to notice more things in nature – little elements that we would not notice otherwise, like patterns on a tree, an unusual bug, a rare plant. Secondly, moving slowly is associated with parasympathetic nervous system activity. The slower we move, the more our bodies believe that we are in a relaxed state, allowing them to slip into relaxation and repair.

Lastly, Amos Clifford, the founder of Association of Nature and Forest Therapy (ANFT), has noted that our pace of walking is often linked to our pace of thinking.[13] Imagine walking somewhere while you are having to make a quick decision about something or are feeling very stressed – many of us would find that our pace increases (and, consequently, we would not normally notice much of our surroundings – to the point that we might even find ourselves somewhere we don't know, wondering how we got there!)

And while many of us struggle to slow our thoughts down (especially if you are a beginner to mindfulness and meditation practice), the beauty of slow walking is that, as we reduce the pace of our walk, we are likely to find that our busy mind starts to slow down by itself.

Our recommendation is to take things slow. If you are a fast walker, we would not recommend immediately slowing your pace right down. Try to first slow the pace down a little bit, then see how you feel and consider whether you might be comfortable to further decrease your speed next time.

How to cope with frustration when slowing down

With forest bathing, as with any other practice, you can only judge what works by trying it. As long as it is safe and you feel comfortable, we strongly recommend you test out each and every practice to find which ones work best for you.

Our recommendation with every practice and exercise is to give it time. Some changes, despite the positive effects that they can bring, can be more difficult than others. Think about changing the pace of your walking or the way you breathe – these are things that we have done a certain way for decades. It is no wonder that when we try to change our usual habits we encounter a bit of resistance. Feelings of frustration or wishing to speed things up, even strong feelings such as anger, are all normal at the beginning of your forest bathing practice and part of the process. Part of being mindful is staying with the emotions and sensations that we feel and allowing them space to surface, acknowledging their presence while not judging them or trying to change how we feel.

With self-compassion and time, we might see that the exercises become less difficult and the emotions are not as intense. However, if you are ever unsure and the strong emotions persist after the practice, we recommend you contact your health care provider to discuss.

As with any new practice, forest bathing can take time to get the hang of. And while the results might or might not be immediate, again as with any practice, the more you do it, the better you become at it (ever tried joining a gym?) The fun bit starts when you begin craving your mindful time in nature and it becomes an established part of your daily self-care routine. That is where we see the most profound changes taking place.

Wear appropriate clothing

There is nothing worse than going for a nice stroll in nature only to discover a few minutes into the walk that you are cold and need to either finish your walk early or risk suffering throughout your whole time outside.

When we are under the canopy of trees, the air can feel moister and cooler than the air outside the forest (even on warmer days). Because we also recommend slowing down while you are practising forest bathing, you might find that it is more difficult to stay warm than during brisker activities, such as a fast walk or run.

Our recommendation is to wear at least a few extra layers on top of what you would normally wear (you can use lighter layers, such as cotton, in higher temperatures, and warmer ones, such as fleece or wool, in colder weather). We also recommend taking a few extra layers with you – you might want to bring a hands-free carrier like a rucksack with you to carry extra clothes in case you need them, and maybe a bottle of water and snacks.

We also recommend wearing or bringing something waterproof, in case the weather changes suddenly. If you do not own any waterproof clothes, you can make a hole in a black bin bag and pull it over your head when it rains. You can also use it to sit down on damp grass if you need a break. There are added benefits to being outside when it rains (see page 125), but they are more easily enjoyed when you are warm and dry.

Shoes with a good grip, ankle support and preferably ones which are waterproof will keep your feet safe while you are enjoying nature. This might mean an investment in hiking boots, but many forest bathers, as well as nature enthusiasts, have found that it is worth it. Good boots, when taken care of, are likely to last years, if not decades, and will keep your feet safe and warm in all weather conditions.

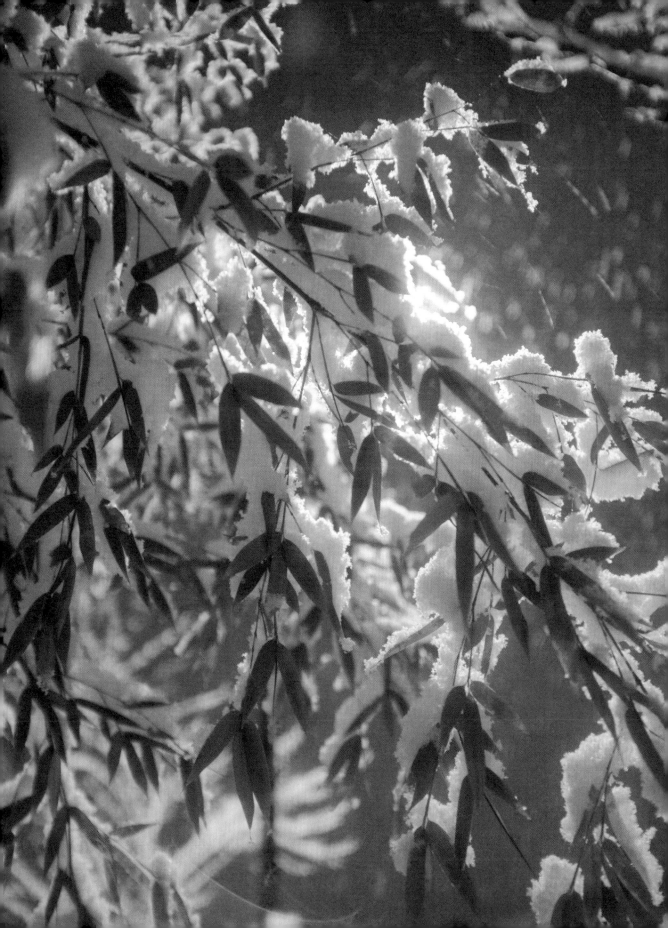

Use your senses and be curious

The only way to connect with the world outside is through our senses. And yet how often do we allow ourselves to do that? How much time do we spend instead taking the information we're getting from the outside world and allowing our minds to use it to tell stories about what it means for us, for our future plans, for our loved ones, for the milk order we haven't yet remembered to cancel?

We recommend that you use your senses to explore the world around you with curiosity and creativity, being open to using senses with which you are comfortable, but also exploring your limits and trying to engage the senses that you don't often use, such as smell or touch. You might be surprised how different your perception of the world becomes once you start engaging different senses!

Many of the participants at our forest bathing events come to our sessions from the local area. Often, the woods that we use for our sessions are the same woods where they walk their dogs, jog or cycle every day. Hence, at the start of the session, these participants claim that they know the woods very well and are intrigued to see if, during the session, they can experience anything that they have not seen before. After the session, the same participants often report feeling as if they have seen the woods for the first time.

When we go somewhere on a daily basis, we often become less curious about the place, for we already feel like we know it too well. The result is that we often lose interest in our surroundings, and with time we notice fewer and fewer details and changes. The same woods that initially brought us a sense of awe lose their charm. But the question we ask you – provided that there have been no major changes in the woods themselves – is this: do you think there is something about the woods that has altered, or do you think the change has come in *how* you look at the woods now, in comparison to that magical first encounter?

In forest bathing, we teach our participants how to bring magic to their perceptions by simply observing what they see, smell, hear and touch. It is, indeed, something very simple, but I can't tell you what transformations it can cause, even in the most sceptical of us. The magic is in simply observing without looking for anything specific, slowing down and staying in the moment, and being open to perceiving what each moment brings you (whether in rain or sunshine!)

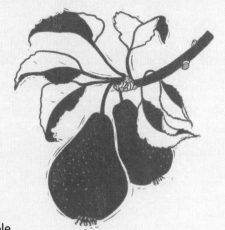

Sensory exercise

For this exercise, you will need a piece of fruit. It could be an apple,
an orange or a piece of dry fruit – any fruit you have handy will do.

1   As you take the piece of fruit in your hand, see how it feels. Is it rough
    or smooth? What is the texture of the skin like? How does it feel to
    your touch?

2   Observe the colours and textures on the skin. Try to notice the
    different colours and shades, and while turning the fruit in your
    hand, observe how the colour changes as the light hits the object
    at different angles.

3   Now bring the fruit to your nose and take a few deep breaths in.
    What can you notice? Does it have a sweet or sour smell? Or maybe
    no smell at all?

4   Slowly take a small bite and give yourself time to savour the
    experience, observing the sensations in your mouth, noticing different
    textures and tastes. Be aware of the sound as you bite into the fruit.

5   As you finish this exercise, take a few moments to contemplate how,
    if in any way, your perception of a piece of fruit has changed while you
    were using all your five senses to explore it. What have you noticed?
    What insights has this exercise brought about?

In this book, we will share with you exercises for different senses, which
you can try to mix and match during your time in nature. If you are able
to stay open-minded and curious, you might find gems when following the
senses that might be a bit outside your comfort zone.

Be respectful of nature and its inhabitants

While you are enjoying exploring nature using your senses, we gently remind you to be respectful of your surroundings. This includes other people using the space, such as walkers, cyclists and horse riders, as well as any animal inhabitants (both small and big) and plants and trees. When you are out exploring, we advise you to only pick up things that are no longer living (for example, rocks, leaves on the ground, twigs) and not to take anything away, as this can impact the delicate ecosystem. If you do wish to pick something up and explore it, our advice is to make sure you place it back either where you found it or as close to that location as is possible. It is important to remember that while for us a walk in a forest can be an exciting adventure, for other creatures, it is their home, so we ask you to treat any natural environment with respect, just as you would another human's home.

This rule applies to all inhabitants of the forest, both animals and plants. When exploring, try to be careful not to disturb animals that might be nesting or hibernating.

It might be best to stick to public footpaths and signed tracks if you are unsure, and/or ask advice from the site manager at the visitor centre, if there is one.

While touching plants can be a rewarding part of a forest bathing experience, we advise you to be delicate when doing so, and also to make sure you know that the plant you are touching is safe to touch (some plants can sting or be poisonous). The same warning applies to using our sense of smell – some plants can produce volatile chemicals that can be toxic to humans (seasonally, or all year round). So, it is best to check first, and if you are ever unsure, enjoy observing the plant, rather than touching or smelling it.

While it is advisable to practise forest bathing in quieter parts of the park or forest, it is still likely that you will encounter other people on your walk (unless, of course, you are on private land). Be respectful of others and make sure you allow them space to explore, while also minding potential dangers from passing cyclists or horse riders.

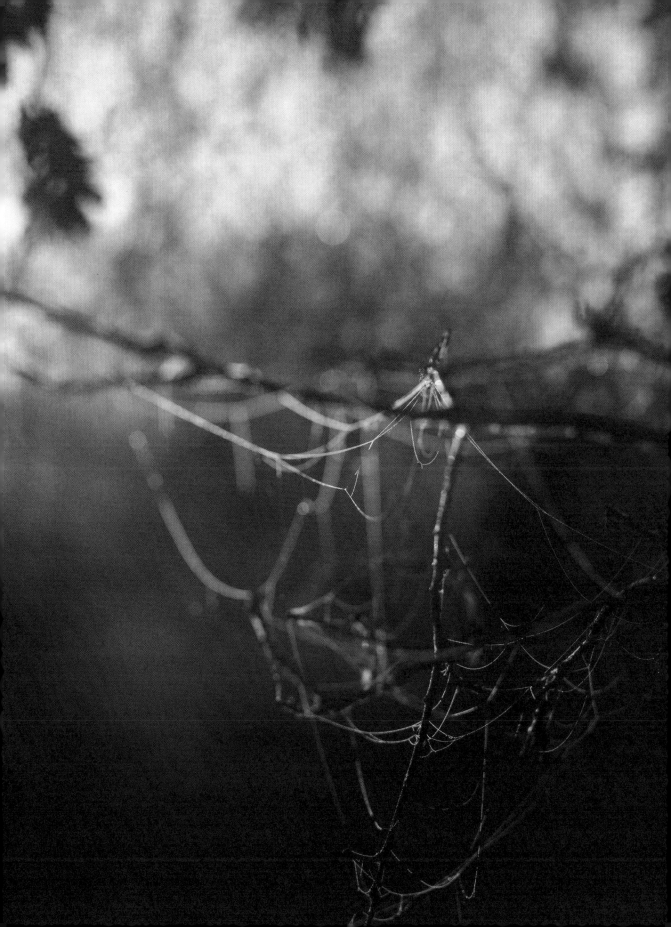

Take deep breaths

Taking in deep breaths throughout your forest bathing walk has a few potential benefits. First, taking in deep breaths is associated with relaxation. It can help us slow down our thoughts and become more aware of the present moment (this is why deep, slow breathing is at the core of many mindfulness practices). Slow breathing can send a signal to the brain that there are no dangers around, which kick-starts our parasympathetic nervous system activity, facilitating relaxation.

Secondly, by taking slow, deep breaths, we are able to take in more of the beneficial chemicals in the air (including phytoncides, see page 59), some of which have been linked to a boost in the immune system.

Slow breathing can send a signal to the brain that there are no dangers around, which kick-starts our parasympathetic nervous system activity, facilitating relaxation

Thirdly, taking in more oxygen helps release endorphins, the 'feel good' chemicals.

We recommend taking breaths in and out through your nose as this allows extra filtration of the air that comes into your lungs. However, you might need to adjust the exercise if you have a cold or hay fever, or struggle to breathe in and out through your nose (which can sometimes take time to get used to, if you are new to it). In that case, you may want to wait until your cold clears, or breathe in through your nose and out through your mouth, if it is comfortable for you to do so.

You should never feel strain in your lungs while taking in deep breaths. If you struggle to do deep breathing while walking slowly, you can start by doing deep breathing while standing still first, and then try to carry on while walking slowly.

If you feel dizzy at any point, we recommend stopping and taking a break. If you are not used to breathing deeply, we recommend starting slowly with maybe 1–2 minutes of deep breathing per walk, and slowly increasing the duration if you are feeling comfortable.

Phytoncides

Professor Li attributes up to 50 per cent of the benefit from forest bathing to the chemistry in the air. In one study, he researched how forest 'aroma', which he created by mixing essential oils from forest trees, affected participants.[14] His findings indicated that exposure to these plant chemicals, together with decreased stress hormone levels, may partially contribute to increased natural killer (NK) cells activity, which are part of the immune system functioning. There are a few chemicals that are produced by the plants that can have a positive effect on human health and wellbeing. Among them, one of the most studied groups are phytoncides. Phytoncides are natural chemicals produced by plants, particularly trees and forests. When released into the air, they have been found to provide several key health benefits.

One of the key benefits of phytoncides is their ability to enhance the activity of NK (natural killer) cells and other components of the immune system. This can help boost your body's ability to fight off infections and diseases. Moreover, phytoncides have antimicrobial properties, which means they can help kill or inhibit the growth of certain bacteria and fungi. Breathing in these compounds may help improve respiratory health and reduce the risk of respiratory infections.

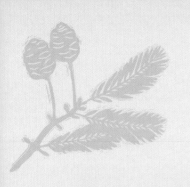
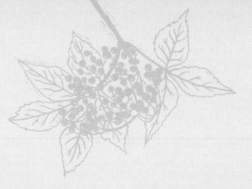
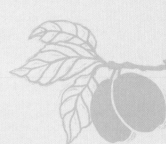

Diaphragmatic breathing — benefits and ways to practise

Diaphragmatic breathing, also known as belly breathing or deep breathing, is a technique that involves using the diaphragm muscle to fully engage in the breathing process. This practice has the potential to help reduce stress due to the stimulation of parasympathetic nervous system, improve oxygen intake as it allows for deeper breaths (which, in turn, can help mental clarity and enhance overall vitality), strengthen and improve the flexibility of the muscles involved in respiration, and even help alleviate tension in the muscles of the chest, neck and shoulders.

Make sure that you never push yourself beyond your limit or experience any discomfort when breathing. We recommend stopping the practice and checking with your healthcare provider if you have any concerns regarding your health.

You can incorporate diaphragmatic breathing when practising forest bathing — this will allow you to take in more oxygen and more of the beneficial chemicals produced by plants in a natural environment. Make sure that you are in a clean, non-polluted environment (as opposed to next to a working factory plant or by a busy road) when practising deep breathing, to avoid breathing in any harmful particles.

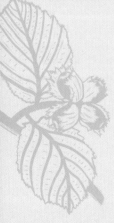

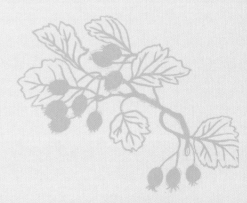

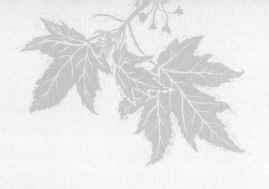
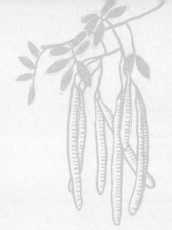

To practise diaphragmatic breathing, follow these steps:

1   Find a comfortable position. Sit or stand in a relaxed position, ensuring that your spine is straight but not rigid.

2   Place one hand on your chest and the other on your abdomen, just below your ribcage.

3   Inhale slowly through your nose, allowing your abdomen to rise as you fill your lungs with air. Focus on expanding your belly rather than lifting your chest.

4   Exhale slowly through your nose, allowing your abdomen to fall as you release the air from your lungs.

5   Continue inhaling deeply and exhaling fully, paying attention to the movement of your abdomen. Try to make your exhalation slightly longer than your inhalation, as this can help further activate the relaxation response.

6   Practise for a few minutes each day, gradually increasing the duration as you become more comfortable with the technique.

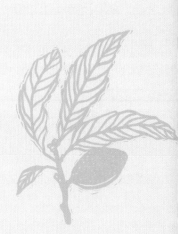

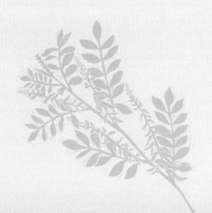

Enjoy the process!

Quite often when we go for a walk in nature, we might already have a route in mind, or a destination that we would like to reach. But with forest bathing, the process is more important than the destination. In fact, the destination has little to no impact on the success of the practice (as long as we stay safe and don't get lost!)

Our recommendation is to start with a shorter route or loop, and instead of aiming to get to the end of it, focus on the forest bathing exercises and your feelings. With practice, you might find that your pace naturally slows down, and you might even want to linger at a spot you like for a while, which is great! Take your time and alter your route if necessary, to make the most out of this practice.

Be mindful of how you feel

One of the big aspects of mindfulness is awareness of how we feel, both physically and emotionally. When you are exploring in nature, ask yourself:

- How do I feel?
- What drew me to this plant/rock/tree?
- How do I feel about this particular colour/texture/smell?
- What made me stop at this spot?

We recommend keeping your questions as open-minded as possible, allowing room for curiosity without judgment and observation.

Often, we assume that we *should* feel a certain way about things; for example, a grey sky should make us feel gloomy, and sunshine should make us feel happy. However, this is not always the case.

Taking our feelings into account and valuing them is crucial to better understand ourselves and our individual needs. The practice of forest bathing encourages gentle self-exploration through contact with nature. And as we explore and connect more with the nature that surrounds us, it can allow us more space so that we might explore and understand ourselves better.

When strong emotions surface

Life can often be challenging. At the same time, with the fast pace of life, we might not always have the time to review how we feel. As a result, feelings of frustration or even anger, alongside other challenging emotions, can pile up without us realizing that they exist.

When we allow ourselves space to relax, it is common for feelings to resurface that we usually suppress or pay little attention to. This can sometimes be a bit challenging, especially if we are not prepared to face strong emotions at the time, or we get surprised by the unexpected appearance of an emotion, or maybe we do not have the resources to deal with the consequences of a strong emotion.

All of this is natural, and only a reminder of how busy our lives can sometimes get.

If a strong emotion surfaces during your time in nature, we recommend taking a few deep breaths to help your body to relax. With practice and if you feel comfortable, you might want to explore what you feel, and why this emotion arose. This can be very helpful in learning more about yourself and your needs, which we can sometimes overlook.

If after your time in nature you feel that a strong uncomfortable emotion persists, we recommend you discuss it with your healthcare provider.

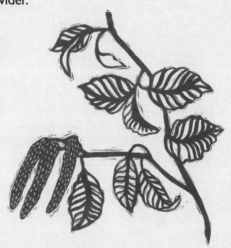

Be kind to yourself and take time

As with any mindfulness-based practice, regularity is key to forest bathing, but another important element to the practice is self-compassion. It is important to be kind to ourselves and to give ourselves time and space to get into the flow of the practice and allow any potential benefits to take place.

We are all individuals and have different lives and different needs. While one person might be able to give an hour every day to the practice and find it quite intuitive, another person might only be able to spare 15 minutes a day and find it a bit challenging as they start. The most important thing to remember is that we are all learning: even experienced forest bathing guides learn every day we go into nature and lead forest bathing sessions.

There is no right or wrong way of practising forest bathing, and any time spent in nature, however short it might be, is better than no time at all. As long as you are not harming others or yourself, and are being respectful to nature and others around you (humans and animals), you can allow your creativity and nature to lead you (and we will share with you a few suggestions of where to begin). Whether you have a few hours or only 10 minutes to spare, if you practise regularly and be patient and kind with yourself, you are bound to see results!

There is no right or wrong way of practising forest bathing, and any time spent in nature, however short it might be, is better than no time at all

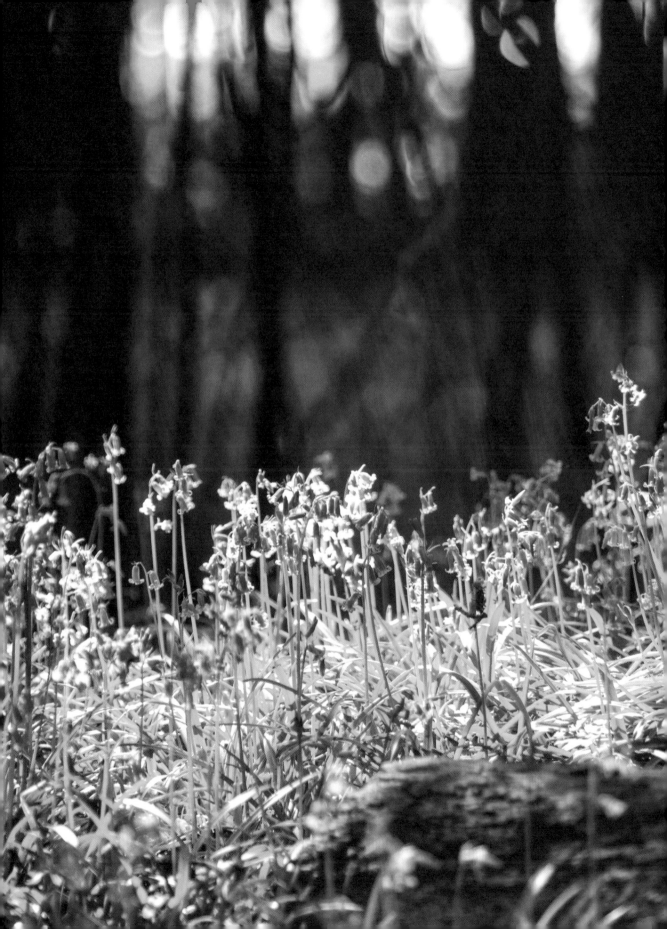

Forest or park: does the environment matter?

While forest bathing originally referred to mindful time in a forest environment, it can be successfully adapted to other environments, including parks and gardens. The regularity and quality of the practice are much more important than where you do it.

If you only have access to a local garden, this can still bring many benefits to you, and the fact that it is convenient for you to visit might encourage you to practise forest bathing more often.

There are some extra benefits to spending time in a woodland environment, and here is why.

A healthy forest environment contains a much wider variety of flora and fauna than parks or gardens. What this means in terms of forest bathing practice is that we get to see many more textures, colours and shapes, smell different forest scents, and we might even be lucky enough to witness a variety of animals if we stay quiet.

Furthermore, as Professor Li has noted, up to 50 per cent of the benefit from forest bathing practice comes from the air chemistry (see page 59). Since forests have greater variety in air chemistry than parks and gardens, we can expect to experience a greater benefit to our health and wellbeing.

Moreover, in a healthy forest environment (unlike in plantations and some newer forests and/or parks), we might find something called the 'Wood Wide Web'. This is a concept developed by Suzanne Simard, Professor of Forest Ecology at the University of British Columbia and the author of *Finding the Mother Tree: Discovering the Wisdom and Intelligence of the Forest*.[15] The term refers to a vast, underground network of interconnected fungi that link trees together in forests.

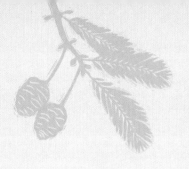
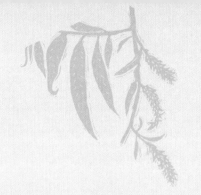

Here's a breakdown of its key features and functions:

- The Wood Wide Web consists of the fungal mycelia which extend from individual mushrooms and form intricate networks throughout the forest floor. These mycelia connect to the roots of trees, forming a mutually beneficial relationship called mycorrhizae.
- Through the mycelia, trees can share nutrients such as carbon, nitrogen, phosphorus and water that might be unavailable to individual trees through their roots alone. This can help weaker trees survive and thrive.
- The network also allows trees to send signals to other trees about environmental changes and threats like insect attacks. Hence, the Wood Wide Web plays a critical role in regulating the health and biodiversity of forests.
- The extent of connections within the Wood Wide Web varies depending on the forest type and species of trees present, and scientists are still discovering new aspects of the Wood Wide Web and its impact on forest ecosystems. But we know that it takes decades to hundreds of years to develop. It can also be easily damaged and broken by soil manipulation and soil compaction, influencing the whole forest ecosystem.

The older and the more undisturbed the forest, the more likely it is to have a healthy Wood Wide Web supporting the health of the whole forest. A healthier forest will be more likely to produce a greater variety of plants and airborne chemicals, protecting trees from invaders and pests and helping to boost our health and wellbeing.

So, if you do get an opportunity to visit a forest, you might want to look for an ancient or semi-ancient forest near you – the older, the better! Consider spending at least two to three hours there, or even go camping – it can be a fun adventure for the whole family, helping you stay in tune with nature and unwind from technology, as well as boosting your health and wellbeing.

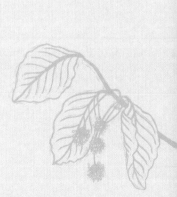

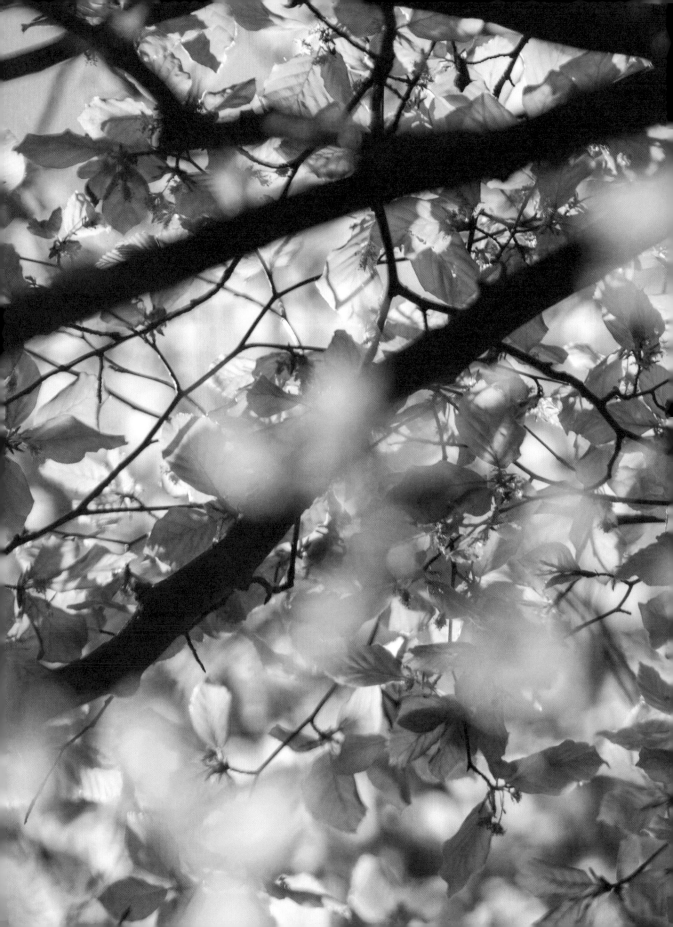

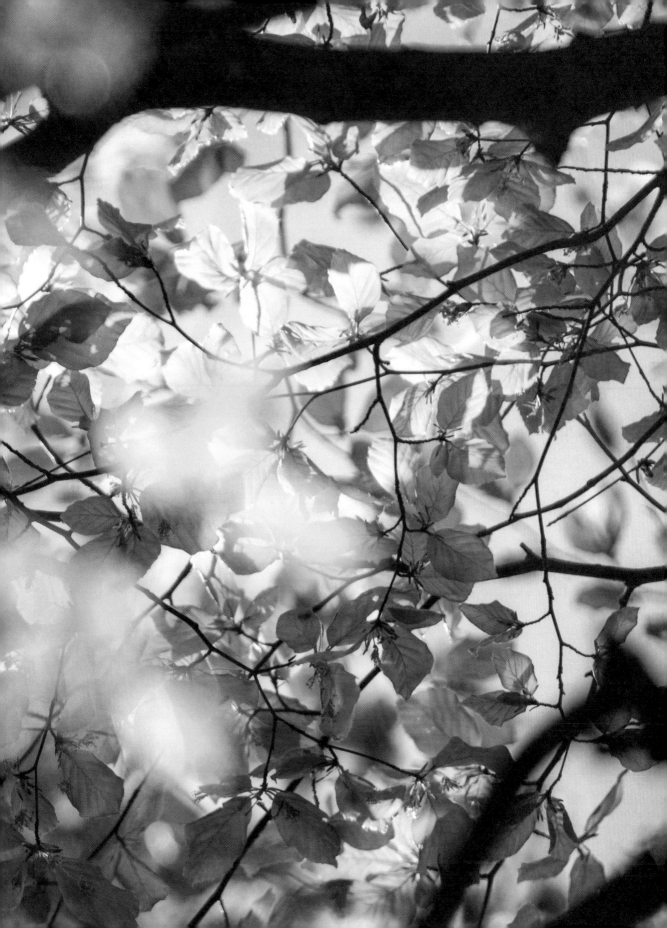

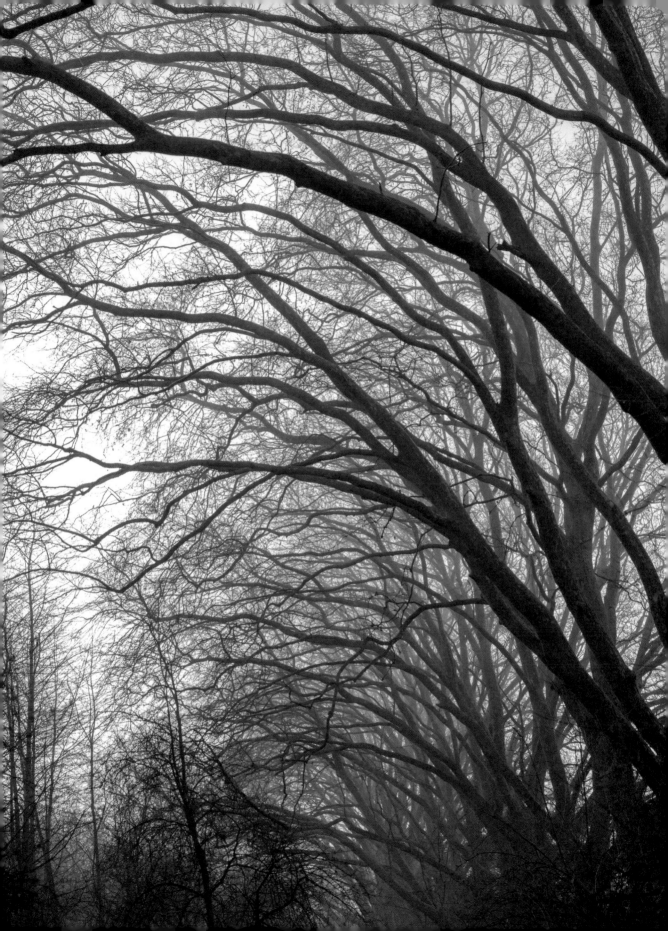

Chapter three

The elements of forest bathing

There are a few elements that are usually included in each of our forest bathing sessions. The main ones that we always try to include are: sensory exercises (for the sense of sight, smell, hearing, touch and, optionally, taste); a mindful relaxation exercise under the canopy of trees – 'treelaxation'; a sharing circle (if you are alone, this can be replaced with contemplation moments); breathing exercises aimed at relaxation, which we encourage you to use throughout your time in nature; and empathy exercises, which are optional.

In this chapter, we will be introducing and exploring these different elements and their role in a forest bathing session. Then in Chapter 4, you will find prompts and helpful tips on how to use these elements to guide yourself through your forest bathing practice.

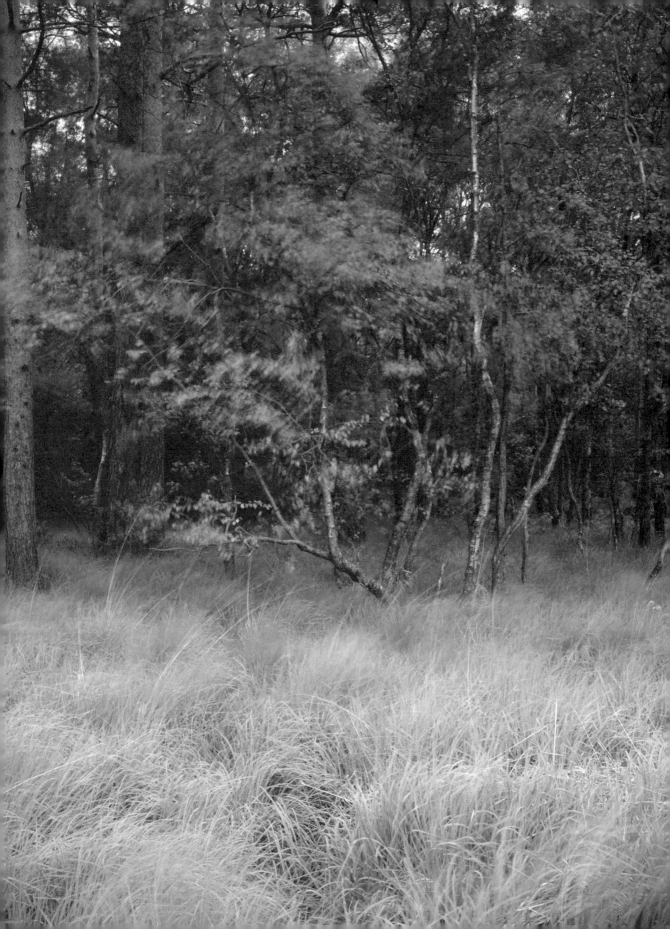

Sequencing

During our forest bathing sessions, we follow a certain sequence of events that seems to work optimally for most people. We normally start with visual and hearing exercises, then move on to touch and smell, followed by optional empathy exercises. We finish the session with treelaxation and a tea ceremony. Slow, deep diaphragmatic breathing (see pages 60–1) is encouraged throughout the session.

In our public sessions, we also have sharing circles where participants have an opportunity to share their experience with others. This is a great exercise to encourage reflection on your experience, as well as to bond with and learn from each other. When practising forest bathing on your own, you can replace this with contemplation and/or journalling instead (you will find some of the contemplation prompts in the sensory exercises in Chapter 4).

The sequence of events you choose to follow in your own practice will depend on a few factors, including the environment, how much time you have available, conditions on the day (including weather conditions, the season,

noise and light levels, how crowded the site is) and your own individual needs and those of others with whom you might be practising. For us, no forest bathing session is identical to any other, and we always adjust our sessions to the individual needs of our participants and the environment.

Below is an example of typical sequencing in our forest bathing practices (each key element will be explored in more detail in the following sections of this chapter):

Sensory exercises: We would normally recommend starting your forest bathing practice with the senses of sight and hearing, which are the senses that we usually use most often in our day-to-day life and are most comfortable with, and then move on to the senses that we are less used to using in everyday life and less comfortable with: touch and smell. However, you might also want to switch things around from time to time as you become more familiar with the practice, and maybe start with the sense with which you are least comfortable.

🔥 **Empathy exercises:** If you are introducing these, they can follow the sensory exercises.

🔥 **Treelaxation:** We always advise a period of 'treelaxation' at the end of your practice. Finishing off your time in nature with a taste exercise, like sipping a cup of herbal tea while enjoying the forest's atmosphere, is often a rewarding experience.

We recommend coming back to mindful deep breathing and introducing some of the breathing exercises (such as 'Mindful breathing' in the treelaxation section in Chapter 4 (page 156)) in between each exercise you do. This will help you further relax and slow down.

The above is a description of a two- or three-hour forest bathing session. However, many of us may not have this time to dedicate to the practice on a regular basis. As regularity is often the key to the practice's success, we reiterate that even 15 minutes of forest bathing a day can be helpful. For shorter sessions, you might only be able to do one or two exercises and may not be able to keep to any specific sequencing.

Finally, we would like to emphasize that the enjoyment you get out of the process is as important as the process itself! As long as you stay present in the experience, it does not really matter much what sequence you use. Indeed, you might want to use the senses as you feel inclined at that moment, following clues from nature – for example, on hearing birdsong, you might start to focus your hearing on it, maybe using some of the techniques described in the next chapter to amplify your hearing. On noticing a squirrel in the trees, you might move your attention to the tree and trace the squirrel's movement across the forest. There is no one right or wrong way to do forest bathing! As long as you stay in the present moment and enjoy the process, you are most likely doing it right.

There is no one right or wrong way to do forest bathing! As long as you stay in the present moment and enjoy the process, you are most likely doing it right

Slow it down

One factor to consider during your sequence of forest bathing events is the speed. As you move through your exercises, it might be helpful to consider mindfully slowing down – not only moving slower, but also going deeper into the details. For example, as you start your practice, you might introduce a few short exercises that do not require too much detailed attention, like simply taking in what you can see around you, focusing generally on colours or textures, or noticing the sounds. After these first few brief exercises, you might want to slow the pace a little bit – instead of noticing any sounds around you, focus on one or two specific sounds; rather than simply looking at your surroundings, focus on just one or two visual elements, like all the different shades of one colour, or the texture of the bark. In the next chapter, you will find suggestions for exercises that will help you make your observations more detailed as you move along the session.

You might also want to physically slow your pace – start walking slower, and by the end of the session, maybe even find a place to stop completely to give yourself time to fully appreciate the forest environment and facilitate deep relaxation.

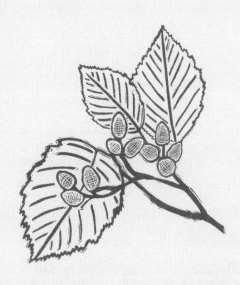

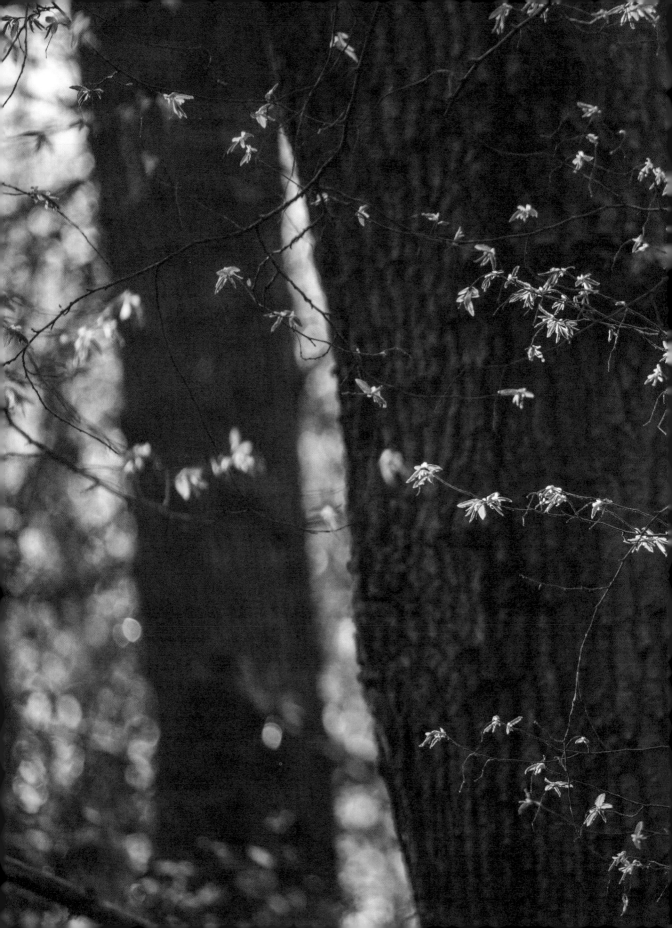

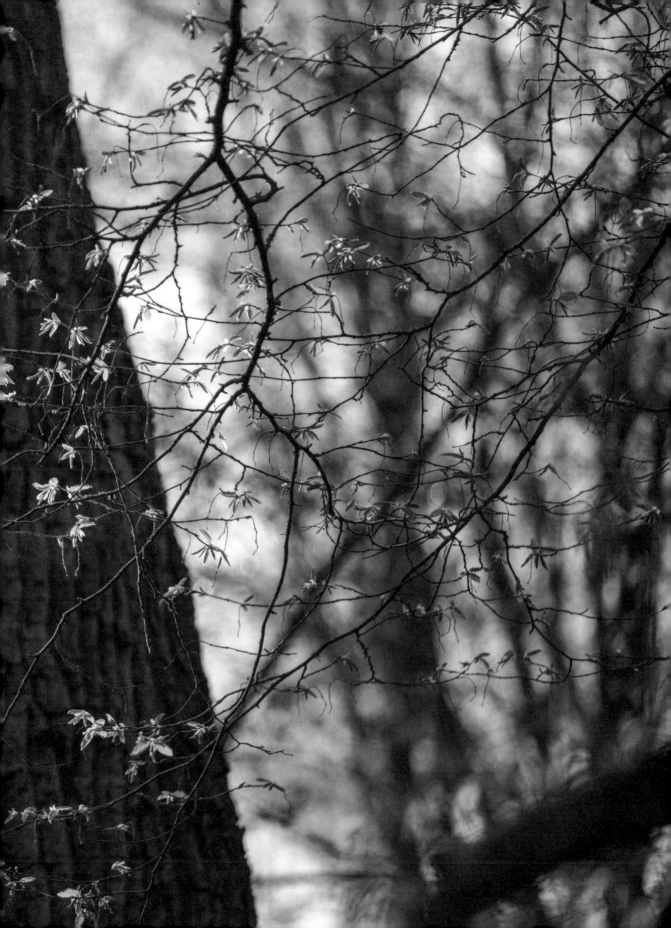

The senses

We have already explained that forest bathing is time spent slowly and mindfully under the canopy of trees, using your senses to connect with the environment around you. Indeed, mindful use of the senses is at the centre of forest bathing practice – but why?

The answer is simple, yet it requires a bit of exploration to truly understand and appreciate the power of our senses.

Senses can be seen as doorways to the world around us. It is our senses that give us information about the world around us, noticing both the hazards and the opportunities that are present. For instance, to understand where you are in an unknown city, you will probably first need to look around to see what surrounds you – maybe, find the name of the street or any major sites that allow you to locate yourself on a map.

When we are in nature, not only can we pick up clues from the environment, but these clues can subconsciously affect our moods and intentions. When we hear birdsong, our bodies naturally relax, because throughout our evolution birdsong has always been associated

with an absence of predators. Similarly, smells can invoke memories of occasions in the past where we noticed the same or similar smells. Smell is a great tool, for instance, for identifying areas where certain edible mushrooms, herbs or fruit might be present.

Not only do the senses connect us with external clues, but they also directly influence our physiology. Have you wondered why certain environments make you feel peaceful and relaxed, while in other environments you may feel uncomfortable, even vulnerable and anxious? This is also due to the way our bodies and minds react to different environments. And while studies have shown that people feel happier in more natural environments than in urban environments (such as a 2013 UK-based study looking at the relationship between participants' momentary subjective wellbeing and immediate environments[16]) there is still research being done into which natural environments are preferred.

As we have been researching the health and wellbeing benefits of spending time in forests, we have noticed that not all forests are the same, and people's reactions to the same forests can vary a lot. While some people might feel most relaxed and peaceful in open spaces with a lot of natural light, such as clearings in the woods, others feel most comfortable and protected in darker, more secluded areas of the forest.

While the reason behind this difference can be due to genetic factors, as well as our upbringing and life experiences, our senses also play a crucial role – both in how we connect with nature through them, and also how we react (both consciously and unconsciously) to the information received through the senses.

After working with thousands of people, we have noticed that there are no two identical reactions to the same sensory exercise during a forest bathing section – each person will focus on something unique and pick out something that resonates with them. And even though reactions may be similar, they are still unique to each individual.

So while the way we connect to nature through our senses and the reactions we have can vary, one thing is for certain – most people feel happier in more natural environments, forests often being high on the list of places where people feel most peaceful.

Discover your dominant sense

Remember the last time you were exploring something? It could have been a new location in nature, or maybe a new object – a present someone gave you. What were the first things that drew you in? The colours, or maybe the textures? The sounds? The smell?

If you have no recollection of the last time you explored something new with your senses, you can pick up an object now (it does not need to be new – it could be something you do not use regularly). Try to notice which senses you are naturally drawn to when exploring an object.

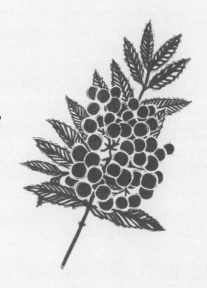

Empathy

Empathy is the ability to understand and share the feelings of another. It involves recognizing and being sensitive to the emotions that others are experiencing, and it often leads to compassionate and supportive responses. Empathy can help build stronger relationships and improve communication by allowing individuals to connect on a deeper emotional level. It also plays a major role in social and organizational structures, fostering kindness, understanding and cooperation in both personal and professional interactions.

One can feel empathetic to people, animals, plants – any living thing. For many of us, a feeling of empathy towards another human being or an animal, might feel natural. We might be practising it in everyday life when we come in contact with our family, friends, colleagues and pets. Feeling empathy for species such as plants, algae and fungi can be more of a challenge, but is possible to develop with practice and imagination.

Our 2019 study with the University of Derby found that after a two-hour forest bathing session, there were improvements in not only mood, but also compassion. Empathy and compassion are closely related concepts, but they are not exactly the same.

Empathy is about emotional connection and understanding. It involves putting yourself in another person's shoe's and experiencing their emotions.

Compassion goes a step further. It not only involves understanding and sharing the feelings of others (empathy) but also includes a desire to help alleviate their suffering or improve their situation.

Compassion is empathy in action. Once we have empathized with another, compassion then acts like a driving force to assist them. When we can understand better what it feels like, we are more likely to help.

Empathy and compassion towards nature can therefore lead to pro-environmental attitudes and actions. The better we understand nature, the more likely we are to help it and protect it.

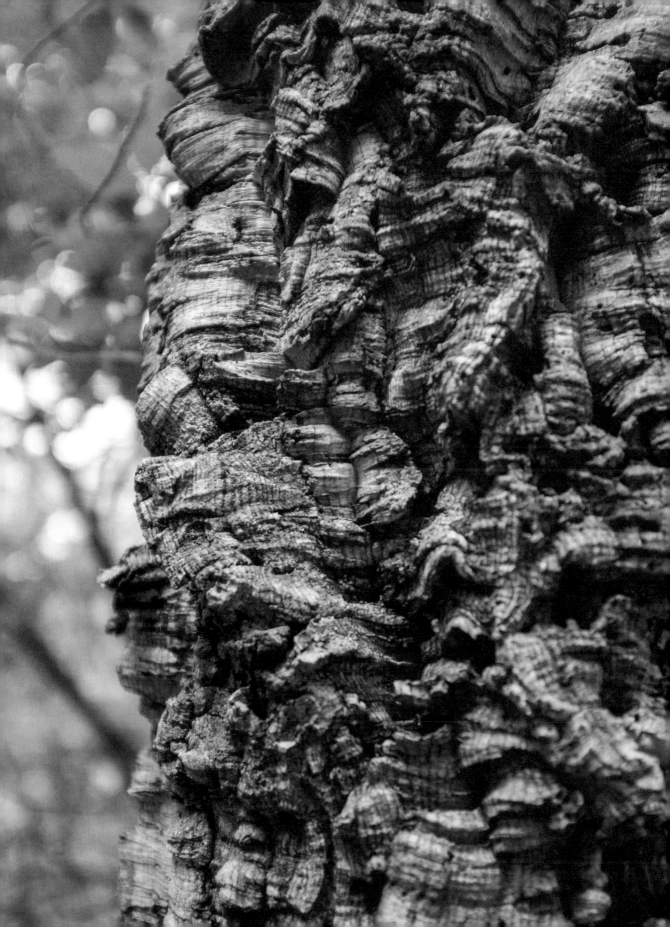

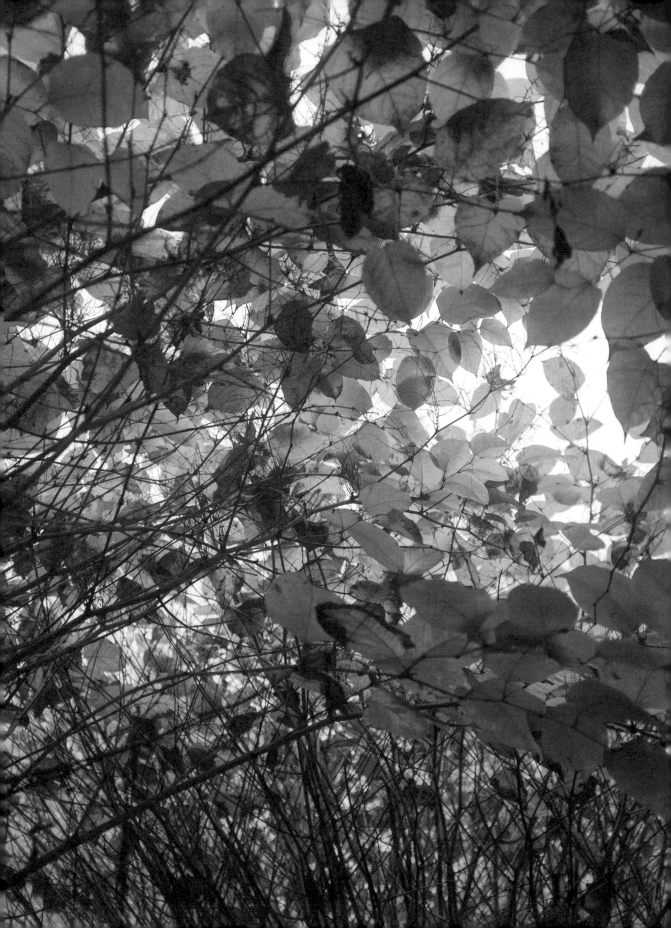

Treelaxation

We often finish our forest bathing sessions with 'treelaxation', a term that combines two words: 'trees' and 'relaxation'. The Woodland Trust, the UK's largest woodland conservation charity, suggested the term to us when we started running our forest bathing events, and we loved it so much that we have been using it ever since! Treelaxation in our sessions refers to lying down under the canopy of trees while relaxing in the forest environment. Our sessions also involve a guided mindfulness exercise by one of our certified guides, which allows you to connect deeper with your senses and facilitate further relaxation. However, you can practise treelaxation by yourself.

Treelaxation is the culmination of our session. Throughout the session, we aim to slow down the pace gradually – we move slowly and also pay more attention to smaller details. In treelaxation, we get an opportunity to stop completely – to simply sit or lie down, enjoying the atmosphere of the forest. Often, a relatively short treelaxation experience can be both rejuvenating and relaxing at the same time.

Some of our participants fall asleep during treelaxation experience, which, of course, is absolutely welcome. However, if you are doing this exercise on your own in the woods, we would advise against this due to safety concerns.

Lying or sitting under the canopy of trees in the forest can be very therapeutic. It can allow us to slow down and appreciate the environment around us. It is often during the treelaxation part of the session that our participants report the most magical experiences – a deer walking very close to the group or hearing a rare bird song. As we stay quiet during the experience, we often encounter foxes, squirrels or other wild animals walking close to us.

Interestingly, this exercise also allows us to feel closer to the forest and that we are part of it. Maybe, this is one of the reasons we often get visited by wild animals during the exercise – they no longer see us as 'out of place' in a forest, and stay relaxed when we are around.

On a physiological level, we can also experience our nervous system going even further into parasympathetic nervous system activity, allowing for more relaxation and healing. No wonder many of our participants report feeling as if they have had a rejuvenating sleep after treelaxation!

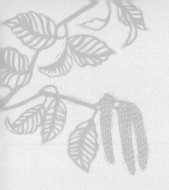
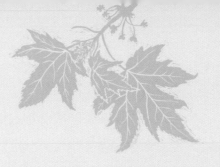
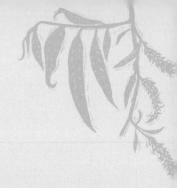

Staying safe

Conditions

🔥 Avoid going outside in high winds (30 miles per hour or higher), during thunderstorms or when there are weather warnings in your area. Check the weather forecast through your local weather service and phone app before going outside, to ensure it is safe and to help you prepare appropriately for the weather conditions.

🔥 We would advise not to go out into nature after dark for safety reasons.

Location

🔥 It is preferable to choose an area in nature where you feel comfortable and safe, ideally not too close to crowded places or busy public footpaths.

🔥 Always check the site you are visiting for safety, as well as for any restricted areas. Some areas might be under maintenance and could be dangerous to visit. You might be advised to stick to the path due to birds nesting or sensitive biodiversity. If you need more clarification, always check with the site management team before going out (in some locations, team management is also available on the site).

🔥 Avoid deep breaths in areas near sources of pollution, such as busy roads or working factories.

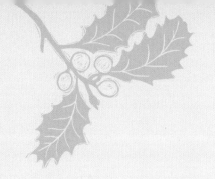
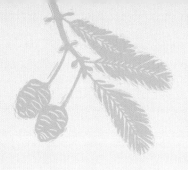
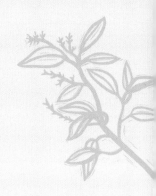

Dressing appropriately

🍃 Always wear long sleeves and trousers when forest bathing, to protect you from insect bites and scratches.

🍃 Dress according to the weather on the day. In warmer weather, make sure to bring a sun hat and sunscreen. In colder weather, layers are essential – you might want to wear two to three extra layers on top of what you would typically wear, as your body temperature can drop when you are in the forest and doing a slow-paced activity like forest bathing. Wear gloves, a scarf and a hat in colder weather.

🍃 If you have them, always bring waterproof layers (trousers and a jacket). You might also want to bring an umbrella.

🍃 Wear sturdy, ideally waterproof, footwear with good ankle support and grip.

What to bring

🍃 Carry any necessary medication with you, such hay fever tablets or an EpiPen. It is also a good idea to carry a first aid kit.

🍃 Carry water and snacks with you when you are in nature. We advise choosing a hands-free carrier bag such as a backpack so that you can freely explore nature.

🍃 Bring a mat (preferably waterproof) or a foldable chair to sit on while in nature. Consider bringing a blanket to keep yourself warm when sitting down.

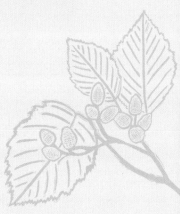

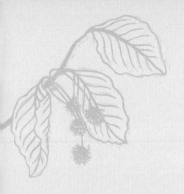

Health concerns

- Avoid touching your face, especially your mouth and eyes, with your hands during your time in nature. Use hand sanitizer and wash your hands thoroughly after spending time in nature.

- Always make sure to check for any sharp objects on the ground before sitting or lying down.

- Ticks and other insects might be a risk throughout the year in some areas. Always check your body for insect bites after forest bathing, safely remove any insects you might find, and treat the affected area. If you have found an insect bite and feel unwell or notice a mark or rash after forest bathing, immediately consult your healthcare provider.

- If you have hay fever, take care when conducting smell exercises and watch for any adverse reactions. It is also a good idea to carry the necessary medication and wait until your hay fever subsides before resuming any smell exercises.

- While forest bathing is a gentle activity aimed at relaxation, it can sometimes bring emotional responses, such as sadness or anxiety. Such responses can be expected as part of slowing down and becoming more aware of our feelings. However, consult your healthcare provider if you feel uncomfortable or the emotions persist after forest bathing.

- Never push yourself beyond your limit. If you feel uncomfortable sensations during forest bathing, such as cold or tiredness, it is best to cut the session short and resume it another time. Immediately stop any exercise with which you are not comfortable.

- If you have an existing health condition or a history of health conditions, we recommend checking with your healthcare provider to ensure forest bathing suits your needs.

- If you are unsure about your health or wellbeing, always consult your healthcare provider.

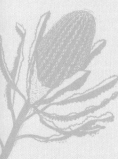

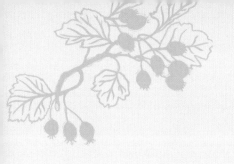

Nature's inhabitants

🌿 Be respectful to other site users and nature's inhabitants, including plants and animals. Avoid making loud noises and scaring animals or hurting plants and trees.

🌿 Avoid touching plants you do not know or are unsure about. It might be a good idea to familiarize yourself with dangerous (for example, poisonous) plants or animals in your area, and the warning signs to look out for, such as skin rash, watering eyes or headaches, after contact with a poisonous plant or animal. If you are ever unsure, it is best not to interact with the plant or animal in question.

🌿 Avoid touching wild animals. If you get bitten or attacked by a wild animal, seek immediate help at your local accident and emergency hospital.

🌿 Do not pick up anything living in nature. Once you have explored objects in nature, return them to where you found them (or as close as possible).

🌿 Beware of hazards such as loose branches that could cause injury.

Solo forest bathing

🌿 If you are forest bathing alone, take a phone with you and let a family member or friend know where you are going and when you are expecting to be back, so they can check in with you.

🌿 If an area is new or unfamiliar to you, be extra vigilant. If you are feeling uncertain, it is a good idea to explore with another person or in a group. Please check the relevant websites or speak to the land management (if it exists) to ensure you know of any recent crimes, accidents or dangers to the public in the area, including which parts of the site are safe to visit.

🌿 Consider staying close to a site's main paths and busy areas, so that other site users are within shouting distance if you need them.

🌿 You can download emergency alert apps on your phone. Should you feel threatened while outside, you can seek help at the push of a button.

🌿 Download the free what3words app on your phone so that your location on the site is easy to identify if you need help.

🌿 Only close your eyes if you are safe and feel comfortable.

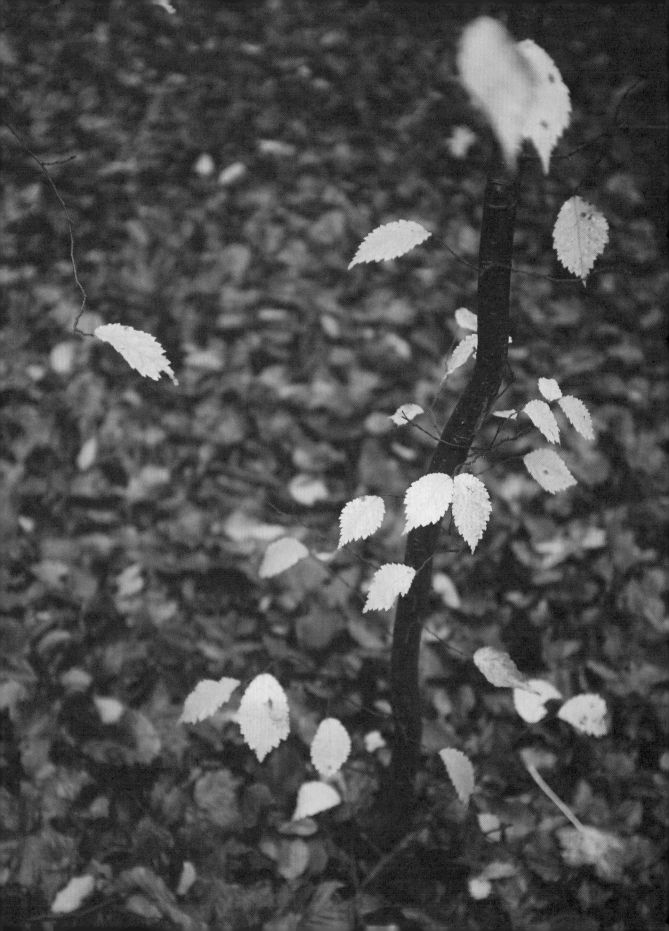

Chapter four

Forest bathing prompts

This chapter aims to provide a practical, easily accessible resource for anyone embarking on a forest bathing session. Forest bathing 'prompts' refer to suggestions or invitations for connecting with nature using your senses. All the prompts in these sections are suggestions only – there is no right or wrong way to connect with nature, and we are all individuals with our own unique needs. One exercise might feel more pleasant or comfortable to you than another, so please feel free to use the ones that resonate best with your current needs (you can always switch things around and try new exercises if you feel like it!)

In the sections in this chapter, you will see forest bathing prompts for different senses – vision, hearing, touch, smell and taste – and also suggestions for treelaxation and empathy.

During your forest bathing practice, you are welcome to mix and match the exercises from these sections as feels right for you.

Depending on how much time you have for forest bathing practice, you might be able to do an exercise for just one sense, or two, three or even four. If you have more time for your practice – for example, if you are doing a two- to three-hour forest immersion – you might even be able to try an exercise from each section. You may find that while longer sessions that use all your senses can bring a more well-rounded experience of nature, shorter sessions where you use your attention to profoundly connect with just one or two senses at a time can be just as powerful or even more impactful. It is all about quality rather than quantity. Your attention, open-mindedness, patience, curiosity and mindful awareness play a crucial role in your practice.

If you find it hard to focus

While noticing various elements in nature can have a great positive impact on our health and wellbeing, it is important to remember that we are all individuals, and what works for one person might not necessarily work for another.

If you struggle with one or more of the senses, choose to focus on another sense instead. As long as you stay with your senses (rather than going into your head and thinking about what happened earlier in the day, or what you are doing afterwards), you can engage with the senses in a way that works best for you and your individual needs.

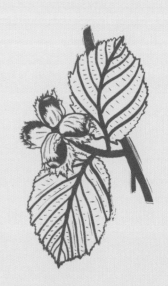

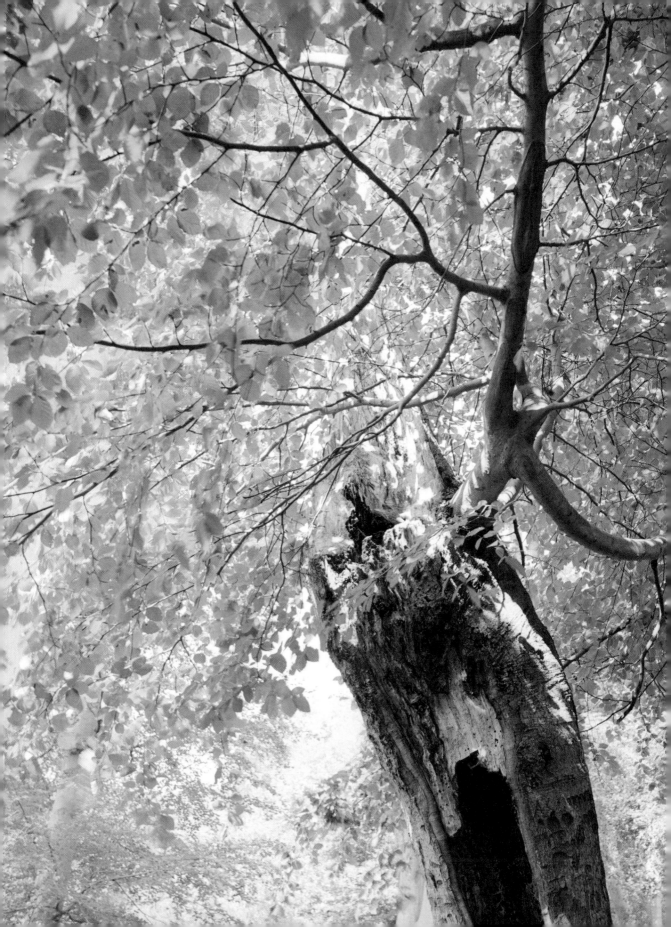

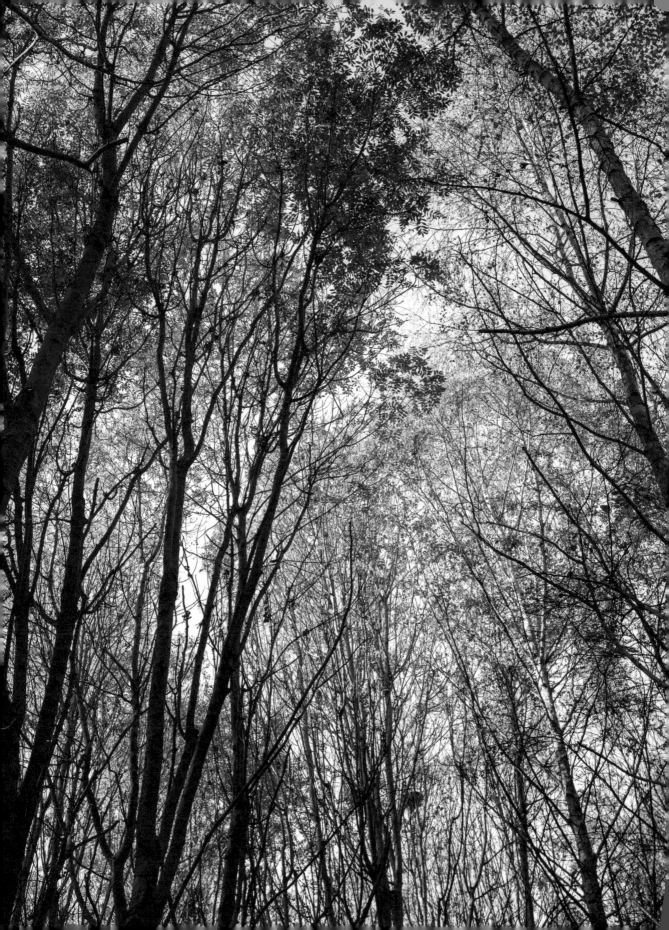

Vision

Engaging with nature through our sense of sight can be very rewarding. Studies show that some of the most relaxing colours are green and blue, which are abundantly present in nature and often forests.[17] Equally, observing different textures and patterns can also have a positive effect on our wellbeing. For instance, studies suggest that exposure to fractal patterns can have positive effects on mental health, cognitive function and overall quality of life. Fractals are complex geometric patterns that repeat at different scales, found in nature, art and mathematics. Research suggests that exposure to natural fractal patterns, such as those found in trees, clouds and coastlines, can have a calming effect on the mind and body. Viewing fractals has been linked to reduced stress levels and improved mood.[18]

Furthermore, some studies indicate that looking at fractal patterns can help improve focus, concentration and cognitive performance.[19] The intricate and self-similar nature of fractals may engage the brain in a way that promotes concentration and mental clarity.

A systematic review of 37 studies into the physiological benefits of viewing nature concluded that looking at images of nature can have a positive physiological effect, and that effect is even greater when we are in nature.[20]

What's more, although this it is not something that can be proven scientifically, we believe that viewing nature is good for the soul. From our forest bathing practice, we have learned that beauty is everywhere in the natural world. We only need to know where (or rather, how) to look. A blade of grass, a little pebble, bark on a tree – through forest bathing, with mindful awareness, you can suddenly notice details that you missed before and appreciate the hidden beauty in the most common, ordinary objects. Often, during our sessions, participants share with us that they have noticed certain things for the very first time, despite having visited that same park or forest daily for years or even decades.

Notice shades of colour

Begin by focusing on different colours or different shades of one colour. Depending on the season and your location, you might be able to focus on different shades of green in summer, different shades of yellow, orange and red in autumn, different shades of brown in winter, and in spring notice an array of colours popping up. Don't rush. Pick an area to explore colours. It could be as small as a flowerbed in your garden or a patch of forest floor in a woodland. You can even do this exercise at home, exploring variations of colours on your plants.

Shades of green

Of all the colours, the human eye can distinguish the most shades of green, on which colour this exercise focuses. First, take a few deep breaths and observe all the colours around you for a few minutes. Then start focusing on the greens – notice the shades of green in the grass, on the leaves of the trees, on the ground. Try moving closer to a specific object or area that contains green, such as a patch of moss, and notice the variations of the shades within it. What can you see?

This is a great exercise to do with kids. You can explore different shades of green together and then ask them questions. How would you describe this shade of green? What does it remind you of?

Observe seasonal colour changes

If you pick a spot in nature to regularly observe (preferably on a daily basis) throughout the year and focus on colours every time you visit it, you might start noticing subtle differences occurring on a weekly, sometimes even daily, basis. For instance, one day you might go out and suddenly notice pops of yellow scattered across your lawn – those beautiful first dandelions in spring. Or one day in the middle of summer you may notice how the lush green is slowly starting to turn yellow and then brown; how trees are changing their vibrant green foliage to yellow, then orange, red and brown. Once you become more attuned to minute changes in nature, you feel more connected to its rhythms and more in tune with it.

Capture colours

If you feel artistic, you could bring a sketchbook and colourful crayons with you. Imagine that you are going out into nature to 'capture' all the different shades of colours that you notice and then bring them back to your sketchbook. This could be a very engaging and fun activity for the whole family.

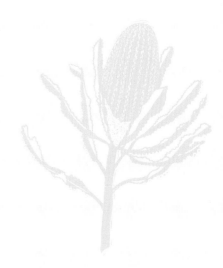

Texture tips

We would not necessarily recommend starting your nature exploration with noticing different textures. This is because, unlike colours, noticing different textures generally requires attention on the finer details. It is therefore preferable if you start your nature exploration by noticing colours, and then after you have explored nature for some time and start feeling a bit more peaceful, move on to noticing textures.

When you notice textures, you might need to get up close. Some great places to explore different textures are the barks of trees, leaves, different plants up close, the ground and different objects on the ground; for example, nuts, seeds, leaves and twigs.

You might want to combine exploring textures with your sense of touch. For example, when you notice different textures on a tree's bark, why not slowly touch it? Do you notice the difference between how the bark looks and how it feels to your touch? You can even close your eyes (if you are safe and feel comfortable) and see if the sensations differ with your eyes closed (see the exercises on page 121).

When exploring more detailed elements of nature, like textures, taking time is of the essence. There is so much to notice in textures, and it can be a very rewarding experience, but similarly, there is much we can miss if we are moving too fast. If you think this is the case for you when exploring textures and you can't seem to notice any differences as you explore, try taking a few deep, slow breaths and then try again.

Observe the texture of a leaf

Find a green leaf that has fallen off a tree. Notice the texture on one side. Is it smooth or rough? Even or uneven? Move your eyes from the centre of the leaf towards its edges and notice if the texture changes. Now turn the leaf over. Is the texture different from one side to the other?

Observe the texture of tree bark

Find a tree that you feel drawn to. Come close to it, standing at arm's-length from it. Pick an area the size of your palm to observe. Move your eyes slowly to notice different textures and colours. What can you see? Next close your eyes, if you are safe and feel comfortable, and take a few deep breaths, breathing deeply into your stomach on an inhale and feeling your stomach falling when you exhale. Slowly open your eyes and observe the same area of tree bark. Do you notice anything you could not see the first time around?

Trace fractals on a tree

Start with a tree trunk and then pick a main branch to observe. Next, slowly follow it as it branches out into a greater variety of smaller branches. Follow each and every little branch as you move along the main branch until you come towards the end of it. You can then trace your eyes back down the branch in the opposite direction, all the way back to the tree trunk.

This exercise can sometimes take a while, so make sure that you find a comfortable spot before you start. You might want to choose to sit on a bench, or maybe bring a foldable chair or a mat to sit on. It can even be very relaxing lying down on the ground on your mat and looking up at the canopy of the trees, tracing the branches of different trees.

This exercise is excellent all year round, but especially in winter, late autumn and early spring when there is no foliage on deciduous trees, as this is when fractals are most visible.

Trace fractals in a sketchbook

Bring a sketchbook and as you trace the branches with your eyes, trace them with a pencil in your sketchbook. When you return home, you can look at your sketchbook to be reminded of your relaxing time in nature.

You can even try tracing your eyes along the branches you have drawn in your sketchbook when you feel stressed or need a bit of a break and see how you feel afterwards. This exercise can also be great if you spend a lot of time on a computer, smartphone or tablet, or if you read a lot. The smooth, slow movements your eyes make while tracing branches on a tree can help them relax and decrease the tension built up from technology use.

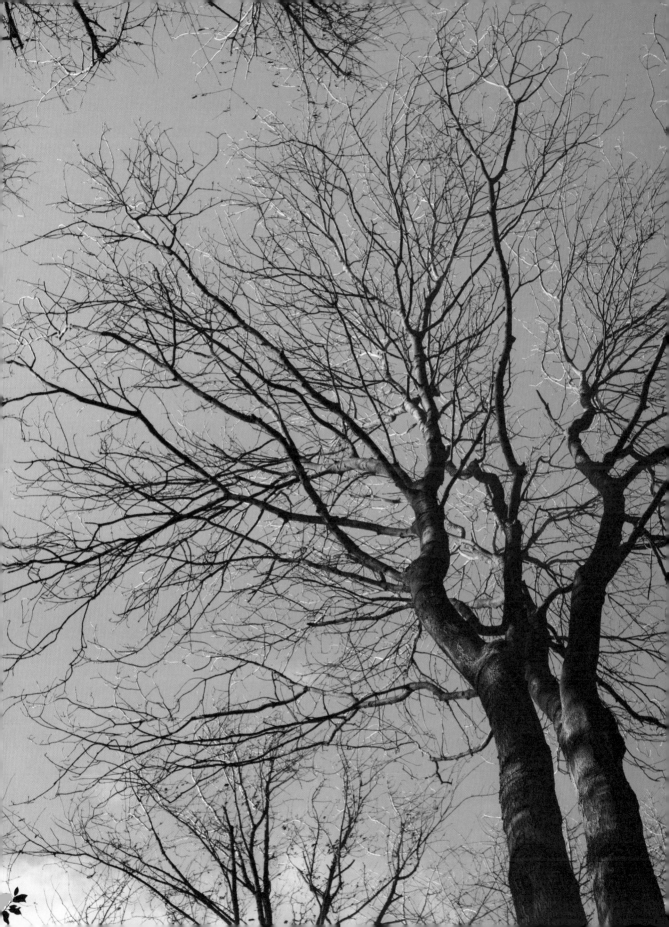

Watch trees in the wind

This exercise is great for spring, summer or autumn when trees have leaves. Find a comfortable spot where you can stay for a while. Our favourite is lying down on a mat on the grass underneath the trees (make sure there are no objects above you that can potentially fall down, like a broken branch). Look up at the canopy of the trees. Observe how the treetops move in the wind. Notice the direction of the movements, the strength of the gusts of wind, and their duration, as well as the gaps between the gusts of wind when there is no movement. Notice how the trees move, or dance, with the wind, how they bend with it. You can focus on one particular tree or a cluster of trees, or even narrow it down to a branch on a tree and observe individual leaves dancing in the wind.

Watch clouds in the sky

This exercise is best done on the top of a hill with a clear view of the sky. If you feel comfortable, lie down on a mat and look up at the sky on a clear day. Notice clouds moving. Now, pay attention to one cloud. Observe how it moves from one point in the sky to another. Notice the speed of movement and any changes in the cloud as it moves – does it grow bigger, or smaller? Are there changes in its shape as it moves? As the cloud disappears, move your attention to another cloud.

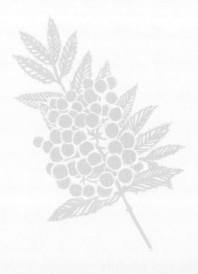

Watch raindrops on the water's surface

For this exercise, you can choose any still water surface – a puddle or a pond is great. Make sure that you come close enough to make out individual drops. Observe the drops land on the surface. Notice the shapes and ripples that each drop makes. What sound do the water drops make? This exercise is great with light rain.

Reflections in a water drop

This exercise is best done on a sunny morning or after a period of rain. Find a water drop on a tree or a blade of grass, in a place where you are comfortable sitting or lying down for a while. Choose a comfortable position to observe the water drop for 5–10 minutes. Start by taking slow, deep breaths in and out through your nose. Then move closer to the drop and see what reflections you can notice within it. Can you pick out any objects or shapes? What colours can you see? If the sun shines on the water drop, notice how the colours change and how the colours of the light are reflected in the drop.

Eyesight

Looking at objects in the distance can help improve your long-distance vision, maintain the flexibility of your eye muscles and reduce eye strain, especially after prolonged close-up work or use of technological devices.

Gazing at the distance can also soothe and calm, helping to reduce feelings of stress and anxiety. Taking a moment to look at the distance can help to clear your mind, improve mental clarity and boost your overall mood.

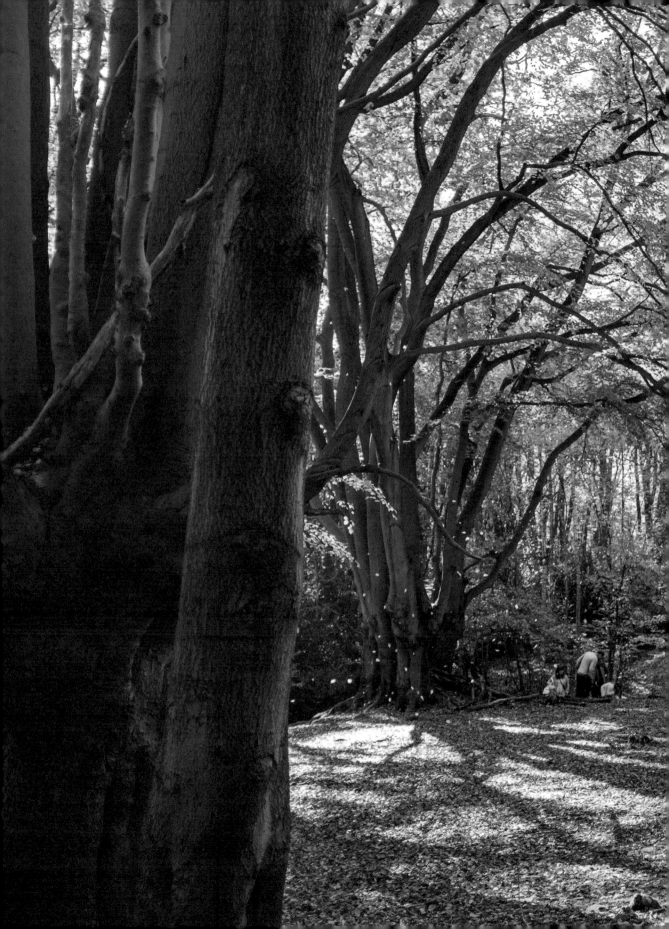

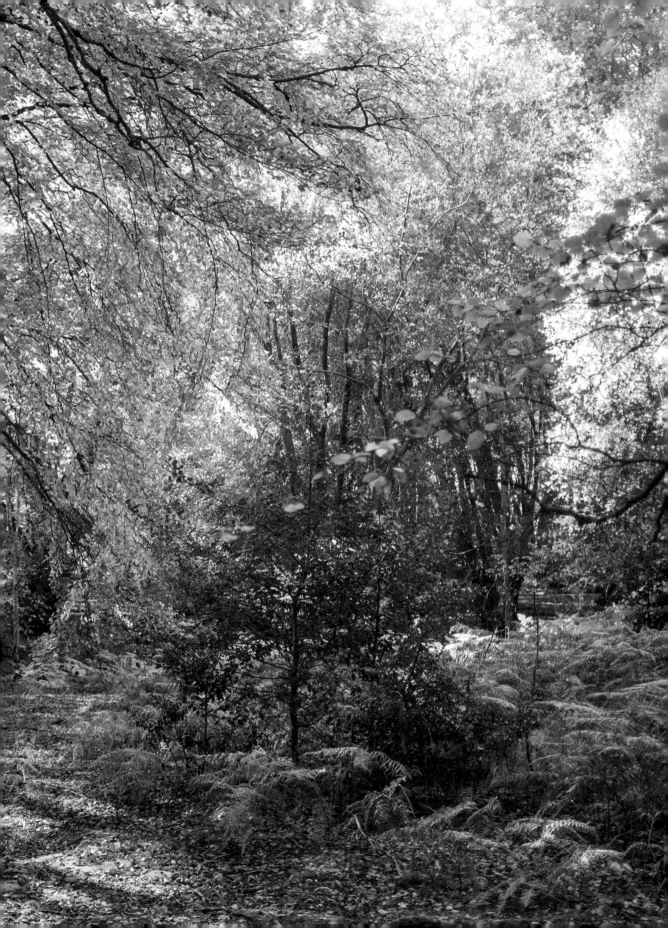

Observe layers

Stand in a place where you can see far into the distance. Ideally, you will be looking at a natural environment, as human-constructed objects like buildings can produce a different effect. Observing fields or trees would be great, but you can also choose to focus on a view of the sea or any other natural water body.

First, find something close to you, something that naturally draws your attention. It could be a rock, a flower, a blade of grass or a slow-moving insect, like a beetle. Focus your attention on your chosen object for a couple of moments. Observe its colours, shape, texture and any movements you can notice.

Then gently move your gaze up to look at something a little further away. It could be a nearby tree, a branch on a tree, a bush, a bigger flower or a plant. Spend a few minutes observing its movements, shape, colours and anything else you notice.

Next, lift your gaze up and look as far into the distance as you can see. Ideally, pick an object or a cluster of objects, like a copse of trees or a particular spot on the horizon. Observe for a couple of minutes, noticing any changes in colours and any movements, and seeing if you can pick out any shapes. At this point, you can also slowly move your eyes along the line of the horizon, noticing any changes in colours or shapes that stand out.

Once you have observed the landscape furthest away, you can slowly start moving your gaze back to the middle distance. If you can, find the object you were concentrating on before and spend a few minutes here, seeing if you can notice any changes in the object this time around.

Finally, move your gaze back to your initial close-by object. See if this object has changed from your initial observation.

At the end of the exercise, close your eyes, take a few deep breaths, then reopen them and take in the whole scene in front of you, with its multiple layers: far away, middle distance and close by. See if your perception of the view has changed in any way from your initial observation.

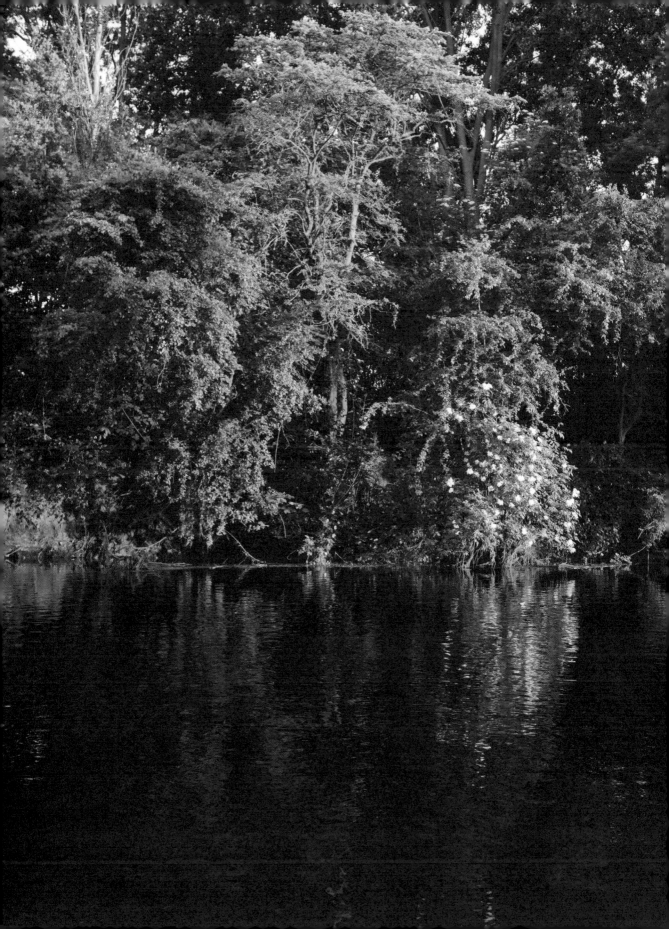

Observe an object mindfully

One of our favourite forest bathing exercises is mindfully observing an object. It does not need to be anything unusual – any object, even the most usual and mundane one, will do – a stone, a flower, a blade of grass. The key is taking time and observing without any expectations.

First, notice one of the colours on the object. What shades can you pick out? Notice how the colours change as the light changes. You can then notice the object's textures – is it rough or smooth? Even or uneven? What is its shape? Does it look different from another angle? You can also observe how the object moves and changes over time – for example, how a blade of grass moves in the wind. Does it look different when it moves?

You can spend anywhere between 5 and 10 minutes on this exercise, or longer if you want. You can also combine the exercise with other senses – for example, touch or smell – and explore the same object using those senses.

Once you have finished exploring the object, you might want to contemplate for a couple of minutes how your perception of it has changed (or not) once you have allowed yourself time to explore it mindfully using your senses.

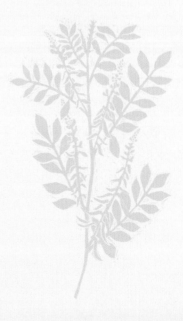

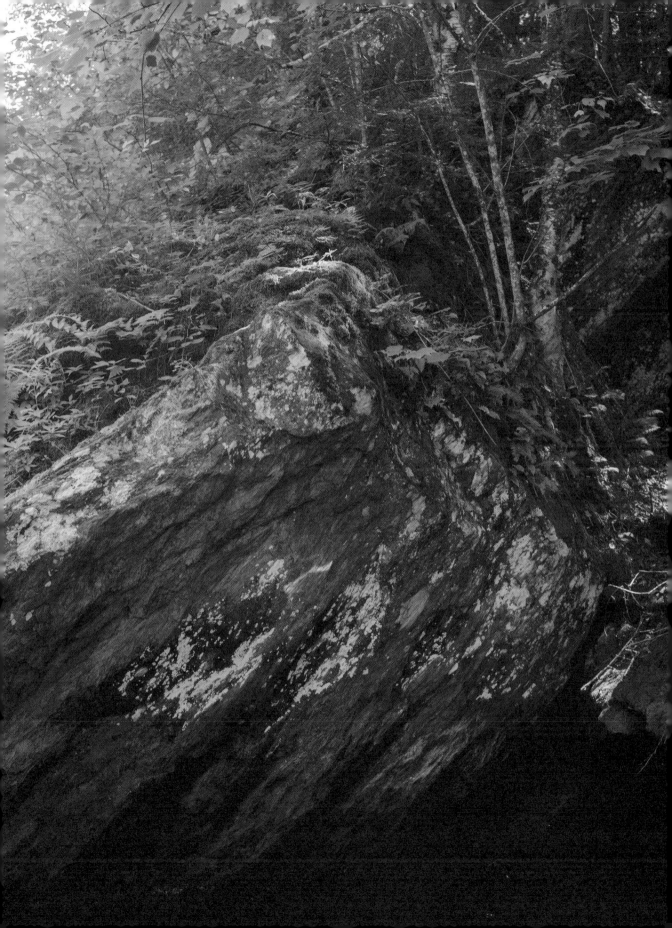

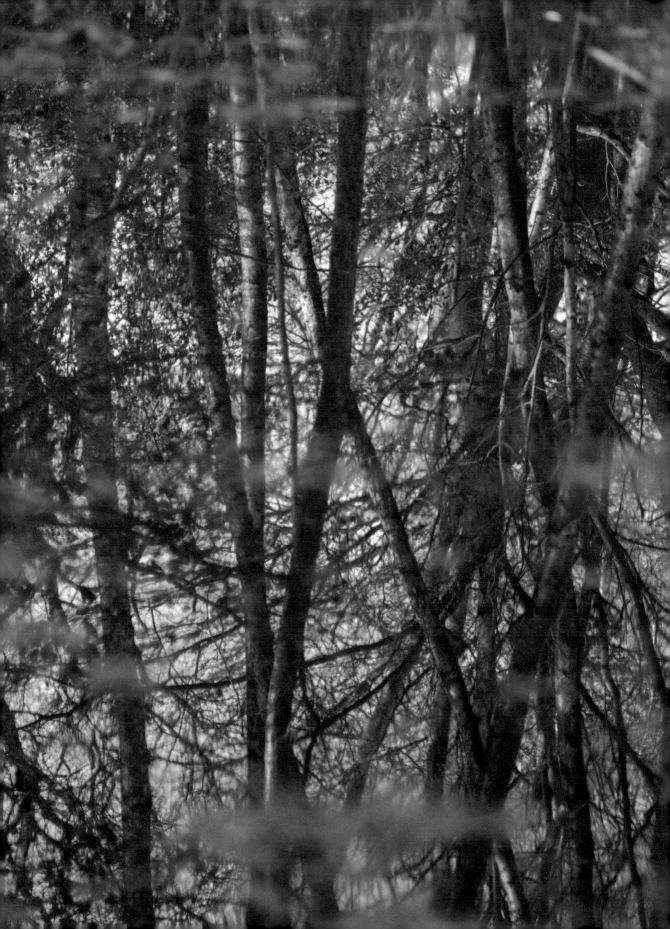

Picture frame

Make a picture frame using your index fingers and thumbs; turn both your hands horizontally, with your right above your left. Keep the palm of your left hand facing you and the palm of your right hand facing away. Then, with each of your thumbs perpendicular to the rest of its hand, touch your right index finger to the tip of your left thumb, and your left index finger to the tip of your right thumb, creating a rectangle. Now direct the picture frame towards an object or a scene in nature – something close to you, like a bush, a tree, a flower, grass or the ground. Observe your chosen scene through the frame created by your fingers. What colours, shapes and textures do you notice? Now slowly move your fingers further apart, expanding your frame. What can you notice now? Move the frame around while expanding it and then moving your fingers back to touching together. What can you notice?

Nature art

This is a fun activity for the whole family. First, find four twigs or sticks to create a picture frame on the ground. You can choose a smooth, clear area or an area that already has interesting objects, textures and colours.

Once you have created a frame, pick sticks, stones, nuts, seeds, leaves – anything that draws your attention. Make sure not to pick up anything living, though. After you have gathered all your supplies, create art on your canvas. Arrange objects in the way that looks most pleasing to you. If you do this as a group, you can take turns adding objects together to create a collective piece of art.

When you have finished, you can take a photo of your artwork (you could even share it with us on our social media @tfb_institute). You can then dismantle the natural art by putting the natural objects back where you found them, leaving the forest in a state as close as possible to how you found it.

Hearing

Hearing is perhaps the second most used sense after vision. It is often one of the first senses we use after vision to engage in our forest bathing sessions.

If you think about how much and how often you use your sense of hearing during the day, you might be surprised. Similar to vision, it often can feel like we are bombarded with sounds from the moment we wake up – the noise of the radio in the morning, the sounds of all the people we are surrounded by as we go about our day, using public transport, going shopping, sharing workplaces, and more.

Noise pollution refers to excessive or disruptive noise that can harm human health and the environment. It is typically characterized by the presence of loud, unwanted sounds that interfere with normal activities, communication and overall wellbeing. It can come from various sources, including traffic, industrial activities, construction work, airports, railways, loud music and noisy neighbours. These sources can produce continuous or intermittent noise that exceeds safe or comfortable levels.

Prolonged exposure to high levels of noise pollution can have a range of negative health effects. These may include hearing loss, sleep disturbances, stress, anxiety, irritability, cardiovascular problems and impaired cognitive function. Children, the elderly and individuals with pre-existing health conditions may be particularly susceptible to the health impacts of noise pollution.

While for many of us it might be impossible to escape noise pollution, there are ways that you can mitigate it and help your health and wellbeing, including wearing noise-cancelling headphones and exposing yourself to the sounds of nature. The latter can be done either through your headphones or, even better, when forest bathing in nature.

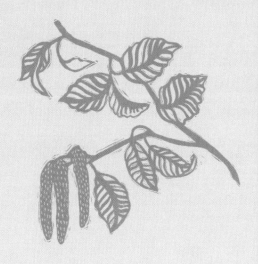

During our 2019 study with the University of Derby, we measured participants' HRV (heart rate variability) throughout a two-hour forest bathing session. HRV readings can often indicate how relaxed or stressed we are, with high HRV generally indicating lower stress. The results demonstrated that HRV readings were highest during three elements of our session: exploring a tree, sharing in a group and listening to the sound of water.

As discussed previously, some natural sounds, such as birdsong, can relax us due to our evolutionary development in natural environments (see page 114). However, another reason for the relaxing effect of natural sounds is the effect of pink noise.

Pink noise is similar to white noise, but is more soothing and smoother. It is a continuous, nondescript sound that combines all the sound frequencies that a human ear can hear. Examples of pink noise include rustling leaves, steady rainfall, running water and the humming of some household appliances like fans or air conditioners. Some people also enjoy listening to specially designed pink noise tracks for relaxation, concentration or masking other unwanted noises. Research into pink sounds, and why we find some natural sounds especially soothing, is ongoing. It is important to note, though, that we are all individuals, with different perceptions of sounds (and, for that matter, different perceptions of other senses too). What one person might find relaxing, another might find jarring or even scary. We can also have different perceptions of the volume of sounds, which will also impact our experience of them.

Despite that, most people find the sounds of nature relaxing. If you find that a particular sound feels more relaxing to you than another, you can focus on that specific one. Otherwise, you can experiment by exploring different sounds around you whenever you are in nature.

Notice the sounds around you

Take a few deep breaths and start paying attention to the sounds you hear around you. Try not to name the sounds or understand where they are coming from – simply allow yourself to bathe in them, noticing as they come and go, as well as the gaps in between the sounds. Can you notice the sounds closer to you, like the sound of your breath? What is the furthest sound you can pick out?

Listen to the rain on the leaves

Choose a spot in a forest or a park underneath the canopy of a tree while it is raining. If you are safe and feel comfortable, close your eyes and focus your attention on the sounds of the raindrops around you. Listen to the sound they make when they fall on to the leaves of the tree above you. Can you hear the sound of the raindrops falling on to the leaves of surrounding trees? How far away can you hear the raindrops falling? When you are ready, open your eyes. How does the sound of the rain change when you open your eyes?

Sound layers

Start by simply listening to the sounds around you as they come and go, while taking deep breaths. Close your eyes, if you are in a safe place and feel comfortable. After listening to the surrounding sounds for a few minutes, narrow your focus to the sounds closest to you – the sound of your breath and leaves rustling on the trees nearby. Continue listening for a few minutes and then move your attention to sounds further away – the sound of trees in the distance moving in the wind, birds and other animals, or running water from a stream you passed a while ago.

Now, move your attention to the sounds as far away as you can hear. Imagine your attention moving out to the edge of the forest, park or city, and reaching even further. What sounds do you hear? Listen for a couple of minutes.

Finally, take a few deep breaths and gently open your eyes. Observe what sounds you can detect with your eyes open for a few minutes.

If you hear human sounds, you can either contemplate the idea that humans are part of nature and observe these sounds blending into other natural sounds, or, if you find them distracting, try focusing on natural sounds. If the human sounds become too distracting, you can stop the exercise and return to it when these have quietened down.

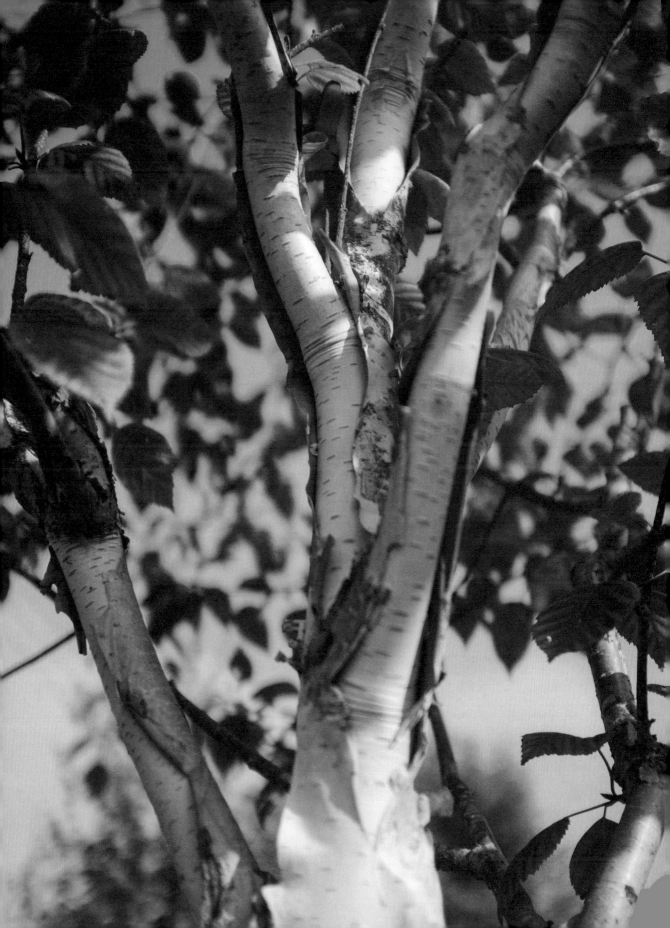

The magic of birdsong

Do you know that one of the theories behind why humans find birdsong so relaxing can be found in our evolution?

Throughout human evolution, the sounds of birdsong have been associated with safety and tranquillity. Normally, when predators approach, we hear alert signals from birds, or birds go quiet. This is one mechanism by which birds are able to pass on danger signals to each other. So when we hear a melodic bird song, rather than loud alarm signals, it indicates that there is no perceived danger around, and our physiological response is to relax.

You might like to combine listening to bird sounds with identifying them. There are a few free apps that help; we recommend Merlin Bird ID. It allows you to identify sounds by sending them to the app, and you can also listen to recordings of different bird sounds in your area.

Trying to identify birds from their song might be less relaxing than simply listening to the sounds without trying to identify them, but it can be more engaging for those who struggle to stay still for periods of time and can also provide a fun educational activity for the whole family to enjoy while spending time in nature.

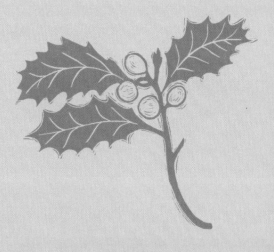

Deer ears

This exercise helps to amplify your hearing and is a top hit during our forest bathing sessions! Cup each of your hands so that there are no gaps between your fingers. Then, gently place your cupped hands behind your ears (for those with longer hair, you might need to move your hair behind your ears first). Gently push your ears forward, just a little bit. Can you notice the difference? You can also listen to sounds in different directions: turn your cupped hands around and place them in front of your ears to listen to the sounds behind you, cup your hands below your ears to listen to the sounds above you (like the wind in the trees and birdsong), and cup them above your ears to listen to the sounds below you (like the sound of your feet moving through the fallen leaves in autumn). You can also try cupping one ear at a time and noticing the different sounds you can hear on each side.

Concentrate on one sound

Close your eyes, if you are in a safe place and feel comfortable, and concentrate on one particular sound that draws your attention. Maybe it is a call between two birds, the sound of the wind rustling the leaves or the sound of the rain. If you choose a spot near moving water, you might want to focus on that sound (a fountain in a park or a stream in the forest is great). Notice the volume of the sound as it rises and falls. If the sound suddenly disappears, notice any periods of silence. What do you observe? How do you feel? You can listen to the sound for just a few minutes or up to 15 minutes – really for as long as you feel comfortable. Then, open your eyes and observe the scene around you. What do you notice?

Listen to the sounds underneath your feet

This is a great exercise for autumn, but it can be done all year round. Choose a path with 'texture', such as a gravel path in a park, or a forest path scattered with twigs and leaves. Start walking slowly, focusing on the sounds underneath your feet as you move. Notice what sounds the gravel makes with each step. Notice the snap of a twig and the rustling of the leaves.

As you walk, you might notice that your path changes. For example, you might move from gravel on to grass. Notice what sounds (or the absence of sound) you can hear now. Continue for 5–10 minutes, or as long as you feel comfortable.

This is a great exercise for kids – you can make it more interactive by asking them to name the sounds they hear as they are walking slowly along the path. What do the sounds remind them of? How do the sounds make them feel?

Record the sounds of nature

The beauty of sound is that you can take it with you wherever you go. For instance, you can record the sounds around you on your phone while visiting nature and then play them back to yourself (or maybe your kids before bedtime) at home, or even at work to help you relax or improve your concentration. You can also get an app on your phone with natural sounds that you like, and listen to it throughout the day. Listening to natural sounds when commuting, studying or working, and before going to sleep can help you to relax after a busy day.

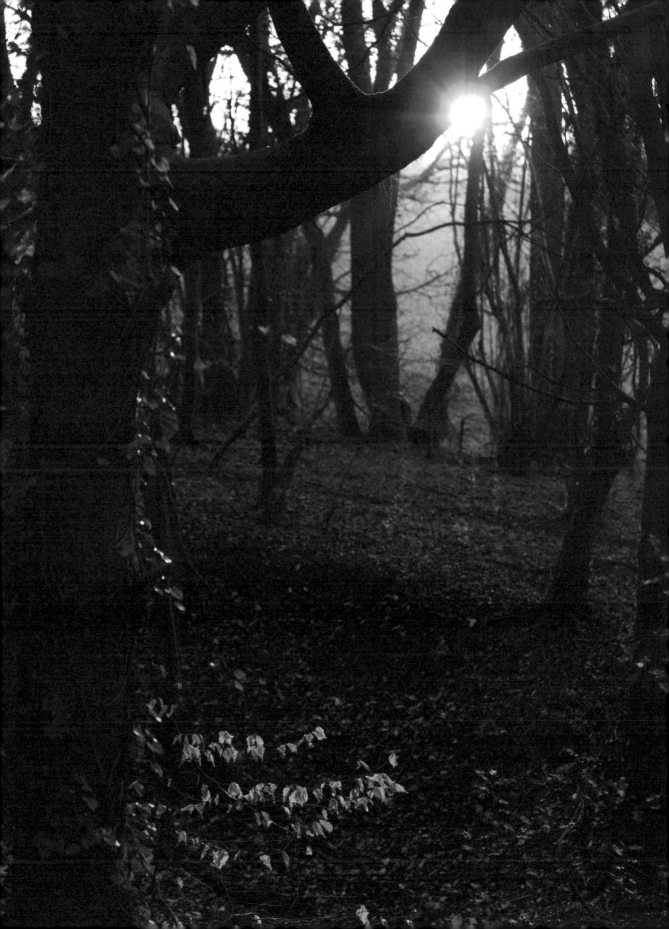

Touch

Try to remember the last time you were aware of using your sense of touch. Maybe it was when you were shopping for a new outfit? Or was it at your local grocery shop when you were picking up fruit? Or maybe it was when you were tending to your plants and checking their soil and leaves?

The sense of touch plays several crucial roles. Touch allows us to feel different textures, shapes and temperatures, which can help us understand and interact with our environment. It also plays an important role in the body's ability to coordinate movements and maintain balance, and provides feedback to the brain about the position of body parts and how much pressure is being applied.

It is also part of our communication with others. Touch can convey feelings, emotions and connection with others through gestures such as handshakes, hugs or pats on the back. It helps to create and enhance bonds between people.

Oxytocin, also known as the 'love hormone' or 'cuddle hormone', is produced when we make physical contact with another human; for example, when hugging or holding hands. It plays a crucial role in bonding between humans, as well as creating trust and empathy. Oxytocin is also produced when we touch nature, and so there is a theory that we can bond with nature and develop a deeper connection to it through touch.

Many find the sense of touch gratifying when we use it to explore nature. Unlike built-up environments, which often have smooth finishes and textures, natural environments have a variety of different textures to explore – from the roughness of tree bark to the plush softness of moss and everything in between.

Next time you are in nature, you can try exploring it using your sense of touch. Find an object that you would like to explore. If it is something big, like a tree, choose a smaller part of it to explore, like a palm-sized area on the bark of the tree, or a leaf on a tree, or a little twig.

You should take a few deep breaths before you start, as it can help your body slow down and become more aware, while shifting towards parasympathetic nervous system activity. You can also start with a few visual exercises first, like observing colours and textures, before you move on to touch, as touch exercises might require more concentration.

You should take a few deep breaths before you start, as it can help your body slow down and become more aware

Move slowly and take your time. Explore the object or area using your fingertips moving as slowly as you can, noticing any differences on the surface. You might even want to close your eyes if you are safe and feel comfortable, and see if the sensitivity of your fingers changes with your eyes closed. You can then open your eyes and compare what you see with what you felt through your sense of touch – you might be surprised at your findings!

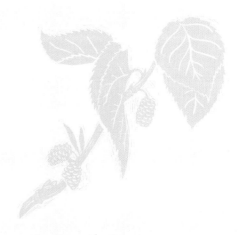

Sensitivity in our fingertips

Our fingertips are especially sensitive due to the presence of a large number of sensory receptors, including tactile corpuscles, Merkel cells and Meissner's corpuscles. These receptors are responsible for detecting touch, pressure, temperature and vibration. The fingertips have a higher concentration of these receptors than other parts of the body, allowing a heightened sense of touch and sensitivity in our fingertips. This sensitivity is important for tasks that require fine motor skills and precision, such as typing, playing a musical instrument or performing delicate tasks with our hands.

A region of the brain called the somatosensory cortex processes sensory information from the skin and is responsible for analyzing touch, pressure, temperature and pain sensations sent from nerve endings in the fingertips. The somatosensory cortex is located in the parietal lobe of the brain and plays a crucial role in our ability to feel and interact with our environment through touch.

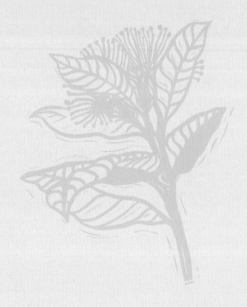

Explore tree bark with open and closed eyes

Standing at an arm's-length distance from a tree, reach out a hand and explore a palm-size area. What do you notice? Now close your eyes if you are safe and feel comfortable. What can you feel now? How has your perception changed, if in any way?

Touch some tree bark

Stand at arm's-length distance from a tree and reach out one of your hands. Pick out a palm-size area to explore. Slowly move your fingers, exploring differences in textures. Does the bark feel rough or smooth? Soft or hard? What's the temperature of the bark? Touch the bark with both hands and see if the temperature is different from one hand to the other.

Explore tree bark using different hands

You can use the fingertips of one hand to explore tree bark and then swap to your other hand. Do you notice any difference in the textures, temperature or the sharpness of sensations in one hand compared to the other?

You can also try exploring using different parts of your hands – for example, see if you can feel the difference between the palm and the back of your hand, or between different fingers. You could even touch the tree bark with your cheek or run a leaf across your forehead. You might find that your sense of touch is different when you are using different body parts, and many people can see a significant difference between the sense of touch in their dominant and non-dominant hand.

Hug a tree

If you haven't hugged a tree before, you might be in for a treat! Choose a tree that you are drawn to. Come up close to it and wrap your arms around it. If you feel like it, and you are in a safe environment, you can close your eyes. Concentrate on the feeling of your body being supported by the tree. How does it feel for your arms to hug the tree? Does the tree feel delicate, strong? Stable, unstable? Warm, cold? You can keep hugging the tree for 5–10 minutes, or for as long as you feel comfortable. After the exercise, you can also contemplate your connection with the tree – what does this tree mean to you? What is the importance of trees, or the forest, in your life?

Trace the veins of a leaf with your fingers

Find a fallen leaf. Hold it in between your palms, feeling its texture and temperature. Does it feel warm or cold? Soft or rough? Then start gently moving your finger, tracing the veins of the leaf. Start at the bottom of the leaf where it attaches to the branch, slowly moving your finger to trace the veins branching upwards and outwards. Once you have reached the edge of the leaf, you can also trace the outline of the leaf with your finger. How do you feel?

You can try this exercise with different fingers, noticing if you can detect a difference in sensations between your fingers.

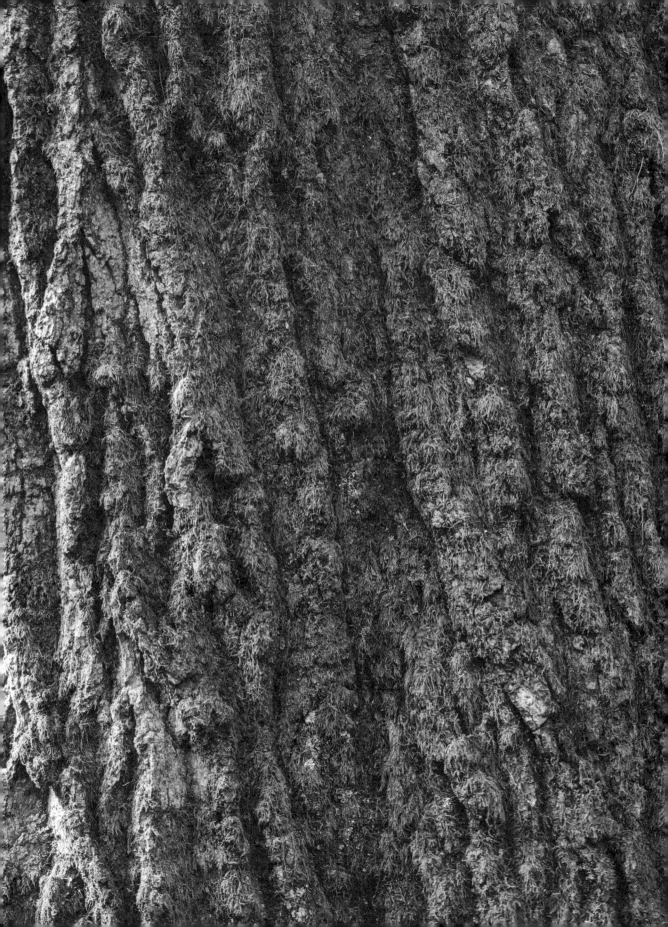

Feel the rain on your hands

When it rains, hold out one of your hands so that you feel raindrops falling on it. If you feel safe, you can close your eyes. Take a few deep breaths. Observe the sensation of raindrops on the palm of your hand. What do you notice? You can then put your other hand out and notice if you can feel a difference between the sensations in your hands. You can also turn your hands over and feel the raindrops on the backs of your hands. What do you notice?

Feel the rain on your face

If you feel comfortable, close your eyes and turn your face towards the rain. Feel the raindrops falling on your face. How does it feel? This exercise is great for lighter rain, but is not advisable during a downpour.

Catch a raindrop

After a period of rain, find a raindrop hanging from a tree branch or a blade of grass. Try to catch the raindrop with your fingertip. See if it remains whole and intact on your fingertip, or if it rolls down or off your finger after you catch it. Observe the sensations on your fingertip as you catch the raindrop. If your raindrop remains intact, take a few moments to observe it before rubbing it in between your fingers. See how it feels to do so, and notice the temperature and texture of the raindrop.

The benefits of going out in the rain

Many of us might struggle with the idea of going outside when it rains. However, unless it is dangerous (we do not recommend going into a forest or a park with winds, or gusts of wind, higher than 30 miles per hour, or during thunderstorms), rain can add extra benefits to your forest bathing practice, for a few reasons.

First, rain increases the amount of moisture in the air, which can be beneficial for skin health, as well as the health of our respiratory passages, helping to keep the optimum moisture level. You might find that in environments with higher moisture in the air, such as during or just after the rain, it is much easier to breathe, and you can even smell more scents in the air.

Second, as rain hits the ground, it releases health-boosting chemicals (which include phytoncides, see page 59) from plant oils that are trapped in the soil and rocks during drier weather. As these chemicals are released into the air, we are able to inhale them.

Third, when it rains, negative ions are produced. These are beneficial for our health and wellbeing, as they knock air pollution down to the ground and also are said to help improve physical performance and endurance, improve sleep and reduce stress. Negative ions, alongside chemicals released from the soil, are thought to contribute to the beautiful aroma in the air during or just after the rain.

Finally, many people find the sound of rain relaxing and soothing. This could be partially due to the random pattern of sounds produced by the raindrops as they hit a surface. As our brain would normally look for patterns, when it is unable to find one, it starts to let go and relax.

Feel the sun and the shade

Find an open, sunny spot where you can comfortably stand for 3–5 minutes. If you are safe and feel comfortable, close your eyes. Take a few deep breaths and focus on the sensations of the bare skin of your face and hands. Feel the sun as it touches your skin, the warmth spreading across your face and hands. Notice how the warmth sinks deeper into your skin, perhaps even spreading to other body parts.

Continue observing for a couple of minutes, while taking deep breaths. Once you are ready, open your eyes. Now, find a spot in the shade. Close your eyes if you are safe and feel comfortable, take a few deep breaths, and once again focus on the sensations of your bare skin. Are these sensations similar or different to when you were in the sun? If they are different, in what way? Continue observing for a couple of minutes and, once you are ready, open your eyes.

Feel the breeze on your skin

Find a comfortable spot to sit down. If you are safe and feel comfortable, close your eyes and take a few deep breaths. Now focus your attention on the bare skin of either your face or your hands. Notice the sensations of your skin. Does it feel warm or cool? Moist or dry? When the breeze blows through, keep focusing on the sensations of your skin. Does it feel warm or cool? Soft or strong? Moist or dry? Continue observing the sensations of your skin as the wind comes and goes, remembering to take deep breaths throughout the exercise.

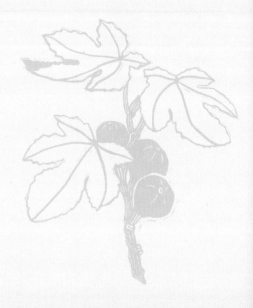

Contrast textures

Find and collect objects with different textures – for example, fallen twigs, leaves, acorns, pine cones and pieces of moss. Make sure to avoid picking up anything living. Spend some time slowly exploring each object using your fingertips, and comparing the experience of touching the different objects. Do they feel soft or hard? What is their texture like? Even or uneven? Rough or smooth? Do they feel cold or warm? When you are finished, put the objects back where you found them.

If you are in a group or with a friend, you can ask them to close their eyes and then present objects to them one at a time, or mixed up together. Ask them how the objects feel, and perhaps to guess what they are. After they have finished exploring, you can ask them to open their eyes and observe the objects to find out if, now that they see them, they resemble the first impressions they received using the sense of touch.

Breathe through your nose

Take some deep breaths in and out of your nose, focusing on the sensations of your nostrils. As the air enters your nostrils, notice how it feels. Is it is cool or warm? Moist or dry? What sensations can you notice in your nostrils as the air enters? Do you feel the pressure of the air being pulled into your nostrils?

As you breathe out, notice the sensations of the air leaving your nostrils. What are they? Are they different to the sensations when you were breathing in? If so, in what way? Is the departing air the same temperature it was when it entered your nostrils? Is it dry or moist?

Kick (or throw) dry leaves in the air

This is one of our favourite forest bathing exercises! When you walk on a thick layer of dry leaves in autumn or winter, if you feel playful, you might want to kick the leaves around and see them flying high in the air. Alternatively, pick a big handful of dry leaves and throw them in the air. Feel the sensations of the leaves in your hands when you scoop them up, or against your feet as you kick them in the air. Watch them fly high and observe how they fall back down to the ground, creating a sense of colourful rain. You can also listen to the sounds the leaves make as you kick or throw them. You might end up with a few leaves on your head, but will create joyful and happy memories.

Put your hands in the soil

Before you try this exercise, make sure you are in a clean environment away from busy paths and roads, and that it is safe to touch the soil where you are (some locations have soil bacteria that can be detrimental to human health). If you are not sure, check with the site's management or on the site's website, if it has one.

Find an area where the soil is relatively soft. Take a bit of soil from the surface layer (you do not need much). You can then gently move it between your fingers, noticing its temperature, texture and anything else. How does it feel to hold the soil in the palm of your hand?

You can also do this exercise when you are gardening, to bring more mindful awareness to the activity.

After you have finished exploring the soil, we always recommend washing your hands thoroughly with water and soap, or if you are outside in nature, you can use sanitizing gel and wash your hands at the next opportunity.

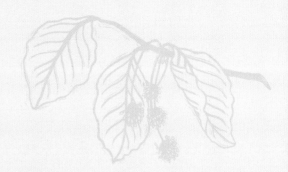

The goodness of soil

Soil contains beneficial bacteria and microorganisms that can improve our mood and overall wellbeing, as well as help improve our immune system and protect us against harmful pathogens.

Mycobacterium vaccae is a type of soil bacteria that has been found to have antidepressant-like effects by stimulating the release of serotonin in the brain. Serotonin is a neurotransmitter known as the 'feel-good' chemical, and its increased production can help improve mood and reduce symptoms of depression and anxiety.

Exposure to soil bacteria can also contribute to the diversity of our microbiome,[21] the community of microorganisms living in and on our bodies. A diverse microbiome is associated with better overall health, including mental health, as it plays a role in regulating neurotransmitter production[22] and immune system function.[23]

Incorporating activities that involve contact with soil, such as gardening, hiking, forest bathing or spending time outdoors, can provide opportunities to interact with beneficial soil bacteria and reap the benefits. Working with it is good for us in so many different ways, including:

- Reducing stress and anxiety
- Maintaining a healthy skin microbiome
- Reducing inflammation
- Improving gut health and digestion
- Increasing energy levels and reducing fatigue

Smell

We are bombarded with different potent smells every day, from fresh toothpaste and shower gels in the morning to vehicle pollution and street vendors.

Natural scents are much more subtle than strong synthetic smells, such as perfume or synthetically scented candles, and when you start discovering natural scents you might at first struggle to pick anything up. However, as you practise using your sense of smell over time, you might be able to develop a better appreciation for more natural, subtle smells.

The sense of smell can be very powerful, as it is linked to our limbic system, which is responsible for emotions and memory. This is why certain scents can trigger strong emotional responses or memories. The olfactory bulb, which is responsible for our sense of smell, is directly connected to the limbic system in the brain, allowing scents to have a strong impact on our emotions and memories.

A smell can have the power to take us back to an earlier time of our lives when that smell was present. During our forest bathing sessions, it is often during the sense of smell exercises that participants suddenly remember moments from their childhood when they spent time in the woods exploring with their family and loved ones.

A smell can have the power to take us back to an earlier time of our lives when that smell was present

Another reason that our sense of smell plays a crucial role in forest bathing sessions is that we can inhale beneficial volatile organic compounds such as phytoncides through our respiratory system, and these have been proven to impact our immune system positively (see page 59).

Lastly, when we smell something and take deep breaths, we can induce relaxation through stimulating the parasympathetic nervous system, which is responsible for rest, relaxation, digestion and healing, amongst other vital functions.

As with the sense of touch, avoid hurting any living things and stay away from poisonous plants. If you are unsure of the species of a plant, it is always best to check or stay away. Some common plants can be highly poisonous, such as yew trees, as well as fern and bracken at certain times of the year when they spore.

Also be aware that the sense of smell is amplified in moist conditions and during or after rain, and you might find it harder to smell during a dry spell. Do not bring things too close to your nose to smell; as a general rule, smell things at a distance of at least 10cm (4in) from your nostrils.

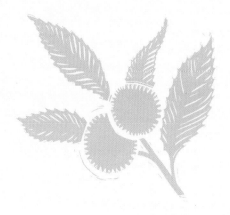

Three deep inhales

For this exercise, find a comfortable place to sit down or stand leaning against a tree. Close your eyes if you are safe and feel comfortable. Take three to five deep inhales, preferably in and out through your nose, although you can breathe out through your mouth if it is more comfortable. With every inhale, notice the cool air coming into your nostrils and down into your lungs. With every exhale, notice warmer air leaving your lungs. Once you finished three to five inhales, open your eyes. Take another deep breath and notice if you can pick out any aromas in the air.

Make sure you do not go beyond your comfort level. If you feel any pain or discomfort, stop the exercise. You may feel a bit lightheaded due to the increased oxygen intake; if this happens, we advise you to sit down and breathe normally for a couple of minutes until the lightheadedness subsides.

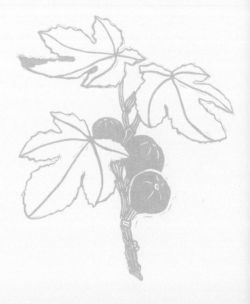

Opening up the sinuses

To help sharpen your sense of smell, you can gently put both hands' middle and index fingers on the area of your sinuses – just underneath the delicate area under your eyes and to the sides of your nostrils. As you take deep breaths, gently pull your fingers to the sides away from your nose. You might feel an opening sensation in your nostrils and cool air entering your nose. You can do this exercise a few times and then take a few deep breaths again, noticing if this preparatory exercise has made any difference.

Three sniffs

Find an object that you can smell – for example, a fallen flower, leaf, twig or pine cone – and see what aromas you can pick out. Make sure to pick up only non-living objects that are already on the ground. Take three to five short, deep inhales (more like sniffs) through your nose. Now try to smell the object normally again. Do you notice any difference?

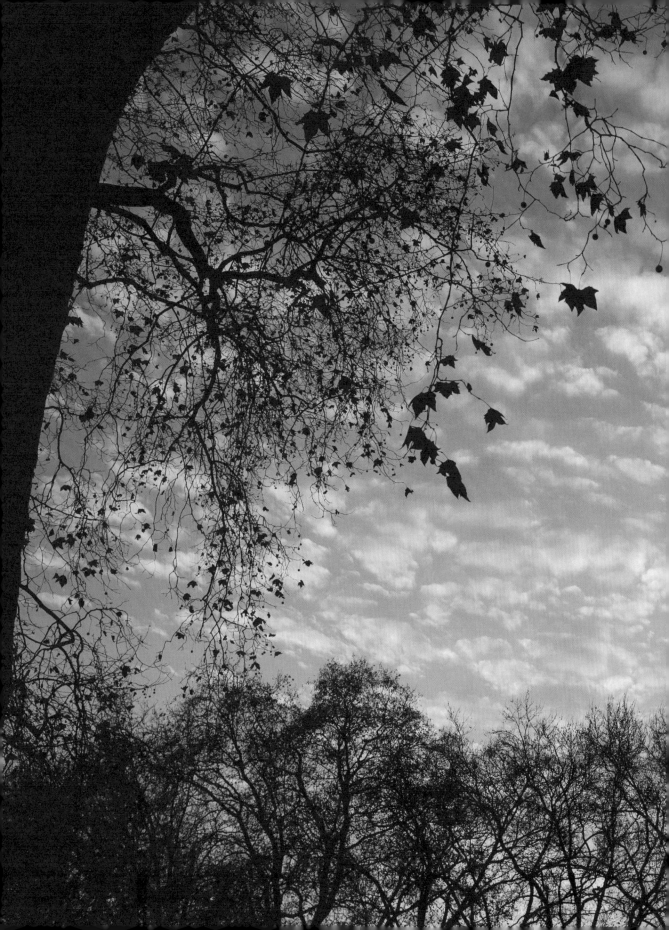

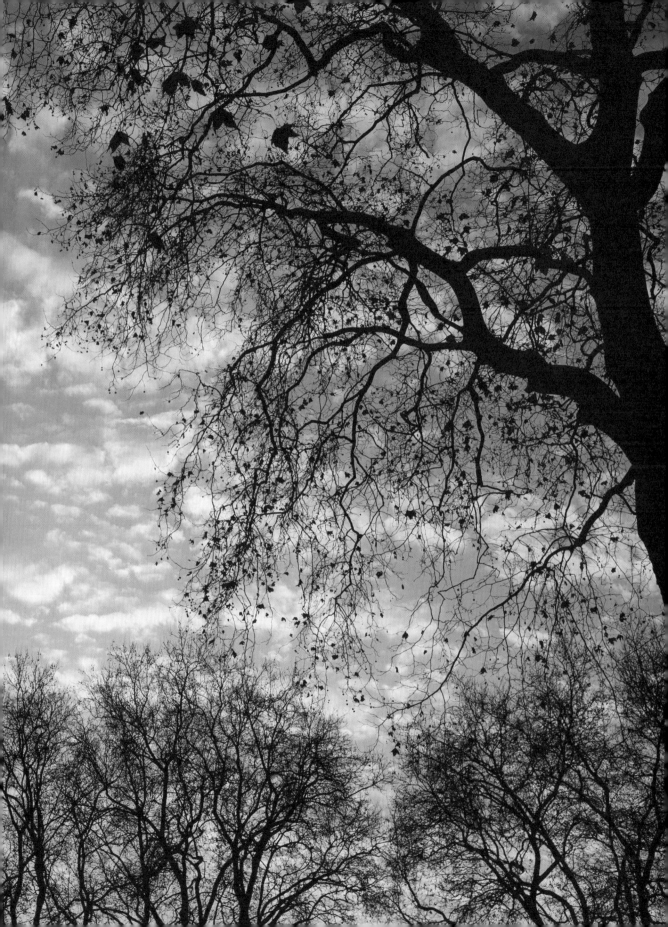

Smell decaying wood

It might sound a bit disgusting, but decaying wood has a very pleasant, earthy smell! See if you can find a decaying log, move closer to it and take a few deep inhales. Can you pick out any aromas?

Smell new growth in spring

In early spring, find new shoots or leaves, or buds on trees. Take a few sniffs and see if you can pick out any smells. If you come across any fallen new leaves, you can also try rubbing them in between your fingers and seeing if they release any aroma. Alternatively, you can smell the new leaves and buds on the trees and bushes – just make sure not to harm any plants in the process.

Smell dry leaves

You can do this exercise all year round, as last year's dry leaves will always be present in a healthy forest. In fact, the older these dry leaves are, the more aromatic they can become. Pick up a few dry leaves and crush them between your fingers. Smell the leaves and see what scents you can pick out. Make sure not to bring the crushed leaves too close to you to prevent inhaling small particles.

Smell green leaves

Find a fallen green leaf on the ground. Gently tear it apart into as many small pieces as possible. Gently bring these up to your nose and take a few sniffs, making sure you don't inhale parts of the leaf into your nose. Our favourites are oak leaves (fresh, or a bit weathered even better!), holly leaves and beech leaves.

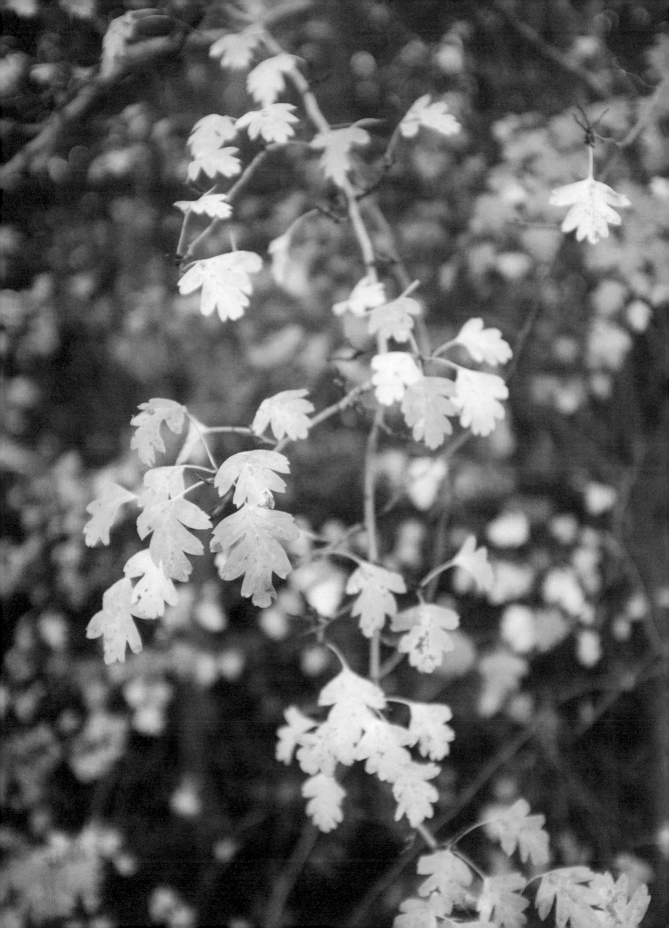

Make a smell cocktail

You can make a 'nature perfume' by mixing together different things you find in nature and then smelling them together. For instance, you might find a fallen leaf, pine cones, pine needles and a piece of tree bark (make sure you don't pick anything that is living). Crunch up each ingredient individually to help release its aroma, and then mix them all together and see what aroma you get.

You can also mix and match your ingredients to create your own personal nature perfume that you can come back to over and over again.

Smell a twig

Find a fallen twig on the ground. Break it into a few pieces and see if you pick out any smell, especially at the breakage area. Now peel off the bark of the twig and smell the twig again, or sniff the underside of the bark. What do you notice?

Smell leaf litter

You can pick up fresh leaf litter in the autumn, or for a more pungent smell, pick up last year's leaf litter by removing the dry leaf layer on the ground and digging up the decaying dry leaf matter (which will, over time, become part of nutrient-rich forest soil). Take a few deep inhales. What aromas can you notice? You might be surprised at the smell you pick out!

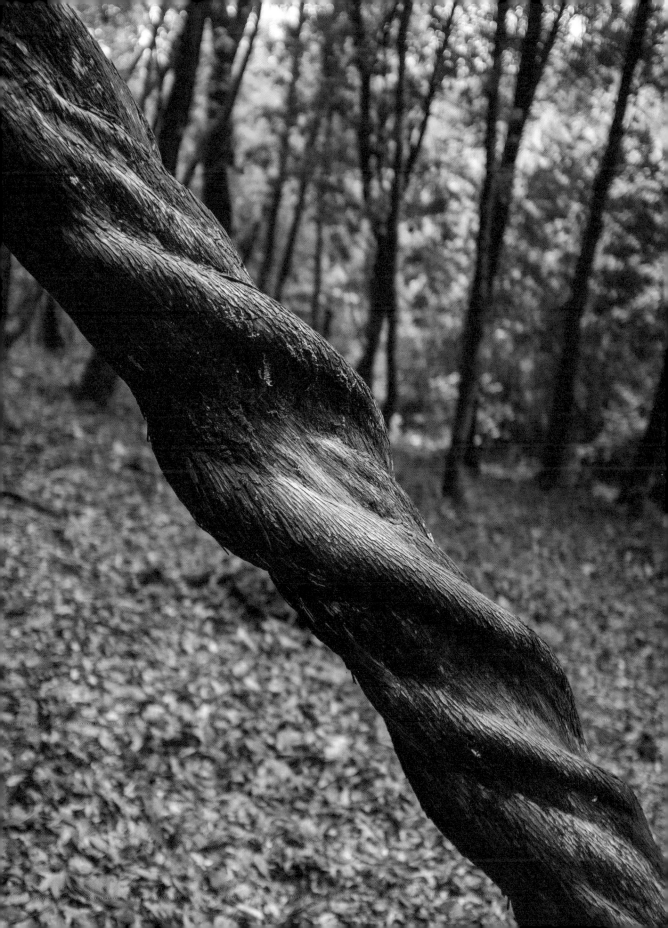

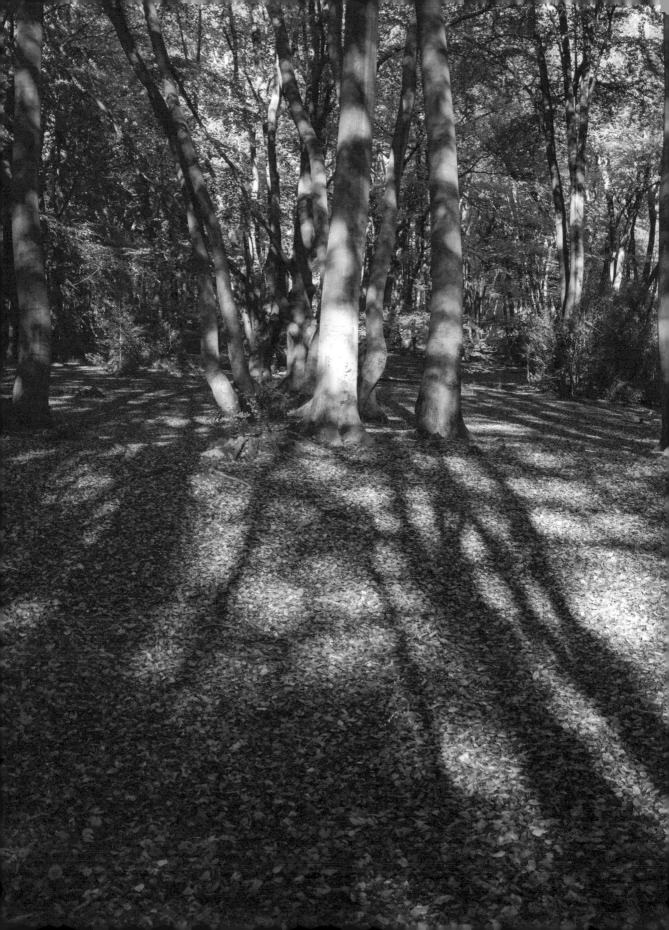

Smell the rain

When it is raining, go out into nature and find a sheltered spot, such as standing underneath a tree. You can close your eyes if you are safe and feel comfortable. Start taking a few deep breaths. Notice the fresh air entering your nostrils and going into your lungs. What aromas can you pick out? How do they make you feel? You can combine this exercise with 'Watch raindrops on the water's surface' (page 101) or 'Feel the rain on your hands' (page 124). Make sure you stay warm and dry, though.

Smell the soil

If it is safe to touch the soil where you are, take a stick and use it to dig into the soil. You may not need to dig deep; sometimes, even a few millimetres will be enough. If the soil is dry, you should dig deeper until you find a moist layer. If you find an area where the ground is soft and/or moist, you might find it easier to dig, and also more aromatic. Once you have dug the soil with your stick, gather some of it on one end of your stick. Slowly bring it to your nose (not too close, though, to avoid inhaling the small particles). Take a few sniffs and see if you can smell anything. If you cannot, go back to the same spot and dig deeper (soil tends to be moister and more aromatic deeper down). Or alternatively, choose a different area where the soil is damper.

If you need it, you can always use hand sanitiser after any exercise.

Taste

You probably use your sense of taste quite a lot. Indeed, most of us have two to three meals a day, and most of us will try to make our meals taste appetizing. Hence, we pay quite a lot of attention to this sense in our day-to-day life.

Tastes are detected by taste receptors located on taste buds on the tongue and other parts of the mouth. The human palate can detect five basic tastes: sweet, salty, sour, bitter and umami (savoury). Taste helps us determine the quality of food, detect harmful substances and enhance our overall eating experience.

Taste preferences drive our food choices, in turn impacting our overall nutritional intake. Certain flavours when tasted can also stimulate specific digestive enzymes, aiding in nutrient absorption.

Taste is a very powerful source of pleasure, triggering the release of dopamine (a neurotransmitter associated with reward and motivation) in the brain. The calming effect of comforting familiar flavours, like a warm cup of tea, can reduce stress levels and improve mood (see suggestions for a mindful tea ceremony on page 144).

Taste can also evoke powerful memories, as we associate certain flavours with specific times and places – for example, a taste of apple pie might bring back memories of summers spent at your grandparents' house where your grandma made apple pie every summer.

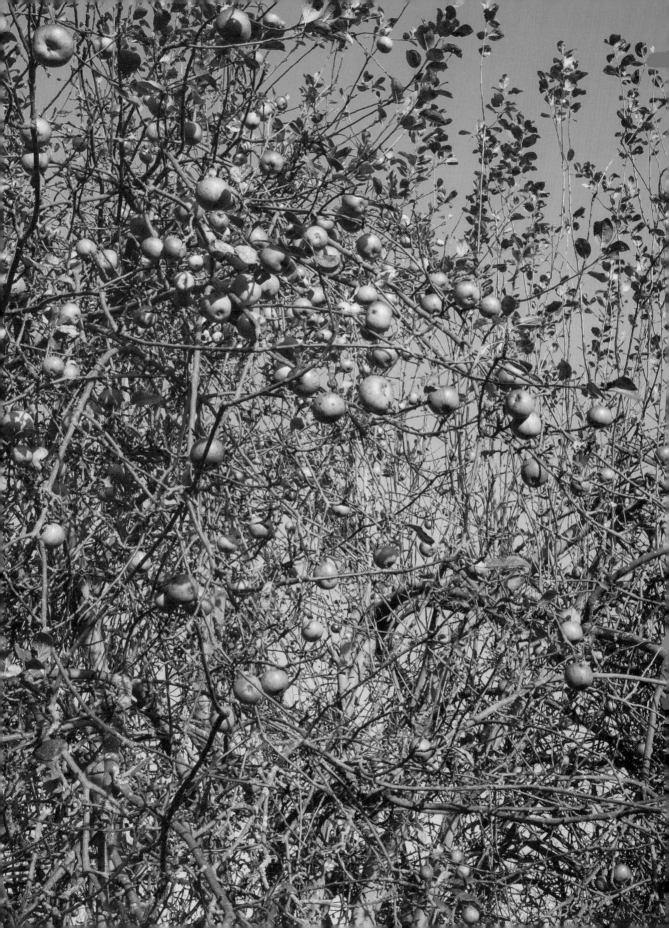

Tea ceremony

For this exercise, you will need to bring a warm drink and cup with you to a forest. You can use any herbal tea (decaffeinated is best) or warm water. We recommend bringing it in a thermos flask to ensure that the drink stays warm.

Find a comfortable spot to sit down. Pour your tea or warm water into a cup. Watch the liquid as it travels from the flask into the cup. Notice its colour, texture and the speed at which it is flowing.

When you have finished pouring, hold the cup in your hands. Feel the temperature of the cup, noticing how it gradually increases as the hot liquid warms it up. What is the cup's texture? Is it rough or smooth? Is the rim even or uneven? Observe the colour and the shape of the cup.

Now, look at the surface of the liquid and watch for any movement, any ripples. What colour is it? Is there any steam rising from it? Can you see any reflections in the liquid's surface? Observe these for a couple of minutes.

Gradually bring the cup towards your nose and take a few deep breaths. Can you pick out any aromas? Feel the warm steam rising from the liquid, entering and warming up your nostrils as you breathe in (only do this if the tea is not too hot, and do not hold the cup too close to your face). Notice how the steam feels as it comes into contact with the skin on your face.

Slowly take a small sip of tea or warm water and hold it in your mouth (make sure the liquid is not too hot). How does it feel in your mouth? Is it warm or cool? Smooth or sharp? Can you pick out any tastes?

Lastly, swallow the liquid (you can close your eyes if you are safe and feel comfortable), and observe how it travels down your throat, all the way down your body. How do you feel?

As you continue drinking, notice every sip and how it tastes and feels. You can contemplate your connection to nature and how each sip you take is part of nature. Or you can feel gratitude towards the Earth for providing you with this nurturing drink, contemplating the journey it has made to reach you today. If you are drinking tea, who grew the plant? Who harvested it? Who helped to get it to you so that you could consume it today?

Picnic in a forest (or park)

Next time you eat a meal or a snack in nature (a piece of fruit works well), try to observe the different tastes you can pick out. Is the food you are eating sweet? Salty? Sour? Bitter? Or umami? Maybe it is a combination of all of these tastes? Try to savour your food, taking your time to chew and explore the tastes.

You can also combine this exercise with exploring using other senses. What colour or colours can you notice in the food? What does it smell like? What noise does it make when you touch it, or chew it? See how the food feels in your mouth. Is it cool or hot? Dry or moist? What is its texture like?

Contemplate the journey that the food has been on to reach you. Where did it grow? Who harvested it? How did it travel to reach you?

Nodate

In Japan, Nodate (野点) refers to a style of tea ceremony that is performed outdoors, usually in a natural setting such as a garden or a field. Nodate ceremonies are typically more informal and relaxed than indoor tea ceremonies, and they often involve elements of nature, such as the sound of birds, the rustling of trees and the scent of flowers. Nodate is believed to have originated in the Muromachi period (1336–1573) as a way to appreciate the beauty of nature while enjoying tea.

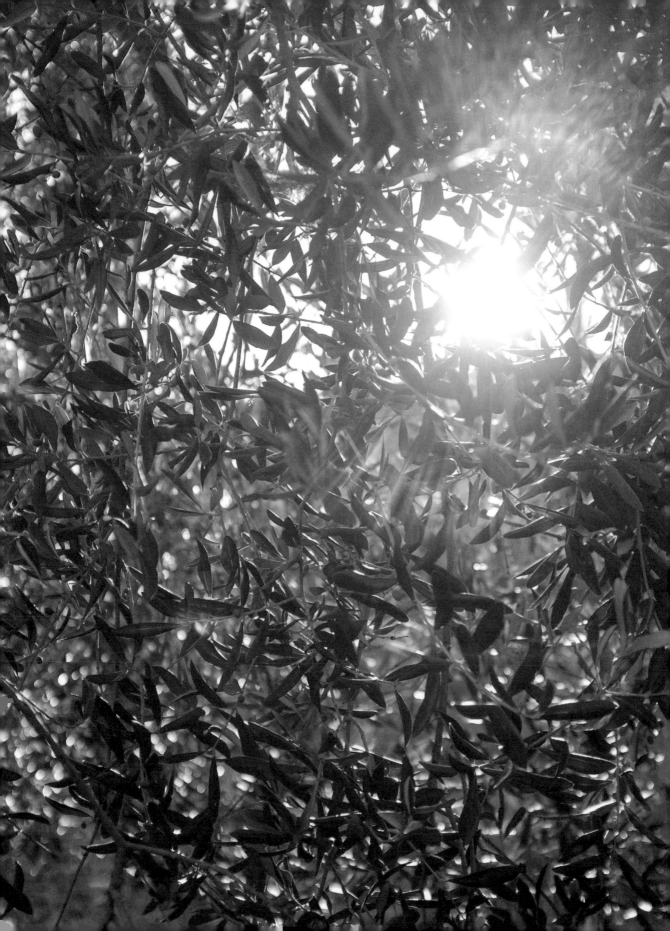

Breathe in forest air

Roll your tongue like a straw, if you can, and take a deep breath through your mouth. You might hear a hissing sound as the air passes through the hole made by your rolled tongue. (If you cannot roll your tongue, simply stick it out instead.) Slowly exhale through your nose, with your mouth closed. On the next inhale, roll (or stick out) your tongue again and slowly breathe in the air through the straw created by your tongue. Notice any sensations on your tongue as you do so. Does the air feel warm or cool? Dry or moist? Can you pick out any tastes that the air leaves on your tongue as you inhale? Slowly exhale through your nose with your mouth closed. Continue for another three to five rounds. Breathe normally and see if you can detect any tastes in your mouth.

This exercise should only be performed in a non-polluted environment and only in warm weather (not during colder seasons). This is because when we breathe in through our mouth, the air that we inhale does not pass through the usual filtration process that occurs when we breathe in through our nose. Moreover, when breathing in through our mouth, we are unable to regulate the temperature of the air coming in (which we can do when we breathe in through our nose).

Taste the forest

Once you have spent a few hours in the forest, lick your lips and see if you can pick out any taste on your lips. You might notice some subtle taste.

Only do this exercise in a clean environment (without pollution), as in a polluted environment, you are likely to get pollution particles on your lips which should not be consumed.

Empathy

Empathy is the ability to understand and share the feelings of others and to imagine oneself in another person's shoes.

Empathy plays a crucial role in our interactions and relationships. It fosters deeper connections with others and encourages compassion by understanding others' struggles. This can lead to helping behaviours, creating a supportive network where people look out for one another.

It can also help enhance our listening skills, making us better equipped to respond thoughtfully to the needs of others, leading to more effective communication and relationships.

Moreover, empathy is a key component of emotional intelligence, which helps us navigate social complexities and manage our emotions and relationships more effectively.

Empathy also allows us to appreciate diverse perspectives and experiences, helping to reduce prejudice and fostering a more inclusive environment. In this respect, empathy can be very useful in helping us build a relationship with the natural world, assisting us in appreciating its beauty and cultivating the desire to protect it.

Mirror a tree

Find a place under a tree canopy where you feel comfortable and safe to stay for 5–10 minutes without interruption, ideally away from crowded places. Look up at the canopy of trees and notice movement. Focus on one tree and, as you continue observing, try to mimic the tree's movements. As the tree moves to the left, move your body to the left. As the tree sways to the right, move to the right. You can even stretch your arms out and pretend that they are branches of the tree. Avoid trying to guess what the next movement might be – simply mirror every movement as it comes. What does it feel like being a tree?

Connect with the forest

Choose a quiet area away from main footpaths. Lie down on the ground or choose a comfortable, safe area to sit down. If it is safe and you feel comfortable, close your eyes and take a few deep breaths.

Imagine roots growing from your feet into the ground. Imagine that these roots flow deeper and deeper into the earth, connecting you with the root system of the trees around you. What does it feel like to be part of the forest, connected to all the trees around you? What role does nature play in your life? What does it feel like to be part of nature? You can continue this contemplation, or imagine your roots spreading even further, connecting you with the Wood Wide Web beyond the forest you are in.

After you have finished your contemplation, you could take a few minutes to write your observations and thoughts in a notebook.

Please note this exercise might not be suitable for everyone. We only recommend it for those who already have substantial experience in mindfulness or meditation, and have done visualization exercises before.

Strike a pose

Choose a tree and observe it for a couple of moments. Notice its shape, how it stands, and its 'posture'. If the tree was a human, what would it look like? Now try to mimic the pose of the tree. Imagine that the tree trunk is your body, and some of its branches are your arms. Adopt a pose that you think most closely mimics the one of the tree.

What does it feel like when you do it? Do you notice any changes in your perceptions of the tree once you have mimicked its pose? This exercise is great for the whole family, and you can take turns mimicking a particular tree – see who portrays it the best!

If you're feeling self-conscious

Empathy exercises are often a big hit among kids, to whom they seem to come effortlessly. However, sometimes we see that adults can be a bit self-conscious about these exercises. Indeed, when you do them for the first time, you can feel a bit silly and childish. But this is one of the points of the exercise – letting go of your inhibitions and expectations and simply embracing being a tree (or a plant)!

Interestingly, many who struggle with this exercise at first go on to report a sense of renewed joy and fun – something that many of us could use more of! Often, these silly-looking exercises provoke deep revelations and contemplations on our place in nature, and foster a sense of compassion towards other beings. What a powerful effect for a seemingly silly exercise, don't you think?

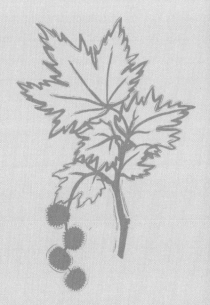

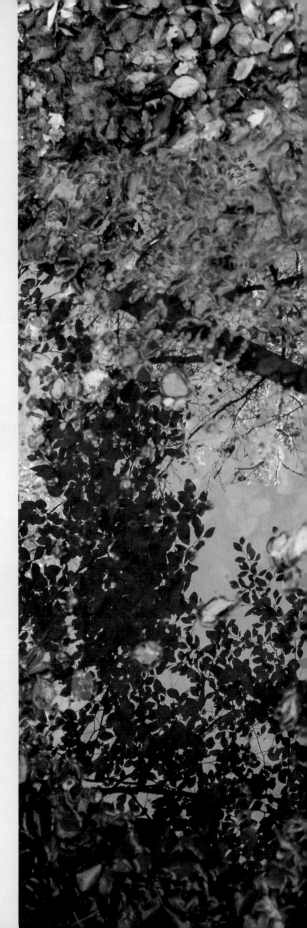

Reciprocal breathing

Find a comfortable, safe place in a clean environment to sit down and close your eyes. Start taking deep, slow breaths in and out through your nose, if you can, for a couple of minutes. When you feel ready, on the next inhale through your nose, breathe in the fresh forest air and the oxygen that the trees have produced. Notice the forest air travelling through your nostrils into your lungs, carrying vital health-boosting natural chemicals. As you breathe out, again through your nose, observe the warm breath leaving your lungs and travelling out of your body through your nostrils. This outbreath carries the carbon dioxide converted by your body back into the atmosphere, connecting it with the forest air, becoming part of it, feeding the trees and plants around you. Continue for 5–10 minutes, or for as long as it feels comfortable. Once you have finished, breathe normally for a couple of minutes and slowly open your eyes. How do you feel?

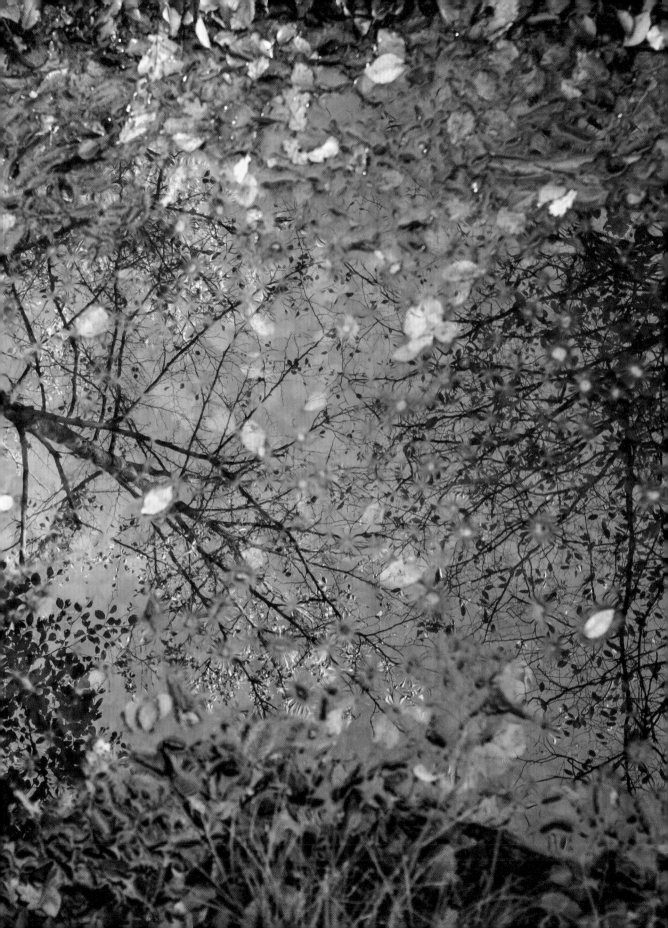

Treelaxation

This exercise is best performed under the canopy of trees; however, you can still do it in a garden with only a few trees.

The aim of treelaxation is to allow us to completely slow down and stop. As we progressively move throughout our forest bathing practice, the goal is to gradually slow our pace, which allows more of our parasympathetic nervous system activity to kick in, facilitating relaxation and healing.

Treelaxation often consists of a few elements, including deep breathing throughout, a body sweep and a sensory experience. There is no one way to practise treelaxation, and you can decide to use one or several elements at a time, but you might experience added benefits if you combine all three elements into one treelaxation.

Normally, a full treelaxation experience would take around 20–30 minutes; however, you can make it longer. After treelaxation, it is advisable to spend 5–15 minutes in silence, if possible. If you brought a notebook or a journal with you, you may want to spend a few minutes journalling your experience.

If you can find an area underneath a tree or trees for this exercise, you can receive extra benefits (and enjoyment!) from the practice. Ensure the space you use is safe and quiet, away from public paths. Choose an area where you have relatively smooth ground (not too many twigs, sticks or stones, so you do not feel uncomfortable). Also, inspect the tree canopy above you to ensure no branches look like they might fall. Check if the trees show any signs of decay or disease, such as insect or fungus infestation, if the health or stability of the trees looks dubious, or if there are visible weak branch attachments. Some trees, such as beech, may not show visible signs of decay or disease but might still be prone to falling. We advise you to take extra precautions and do your own research into trees in the area, as well as check with the site management (if it exists) for safe areas to use. Avoid practising in areas about which you are unsure. If in doubt, choose an area with only one or couple of trees that you are sure is safe to use.

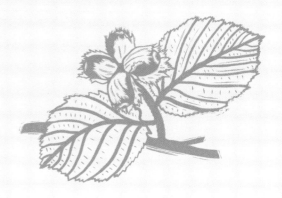

Once you have picked your spot, place your mat on the ground and lie on top of it. Try to make yourself as comfortable as possible – you might bring a blanket to keep warm or choose to put on extra layers. If you feel uncomfortable at any point during treelaxation, you can always change your position.

If the weather is poor and/or you feel cold or uncomfortable lying down, you can always opt to sit on a log or a foldable chair or lean on a tree instead.

Treelaxation often consists of a few elements, including deep breathing throughout, a body sweep and a sensory experience at the end

We would generally advise not lying down in cold weather to avoid frostbite. It also may not be suitable to lie down on the forest floor in some locations and countries due to local flora or fauna. It is critical to understand any local wildlife risks, such as insects or snakes. In the UK, ticks are the main concern, and you should be especially aware if you are in an area with large animals such as cows, sheep or deer, as this increases the likelihood of ticks. Always check any safety issues with the site management and avoid lying down if you are unsure.

If you come to the forest with a friend or a family member and you feel safe doing so, you can close your eyes (one of you should stay with your eyes open, though, for safety reasons).

Mindful breathing

Sit somewhere where you won't be disturbed.
If you can, make sure your back is straight and
your posture is comfortable. Put one or both
of your hands on your belly. Close your eyes
if you are safe and feel comfortable, and take a
deep, slow breath, inhaling through your nose
(if possible), feeling your belly rise and expand.
Then, slowly exhale also through your nose,
feeling your belly fall and deflate. Continue
breathing deeply and focusing on the rise and
fall of your belly for a couple of minutes or for
as long as you feel comfortable.

   You should avoid this exercise if you have a
cold, and only practise it if you are in a clean
environment.

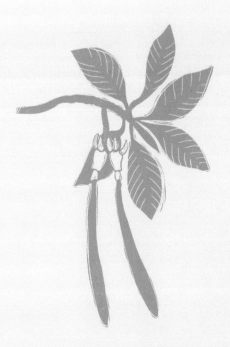

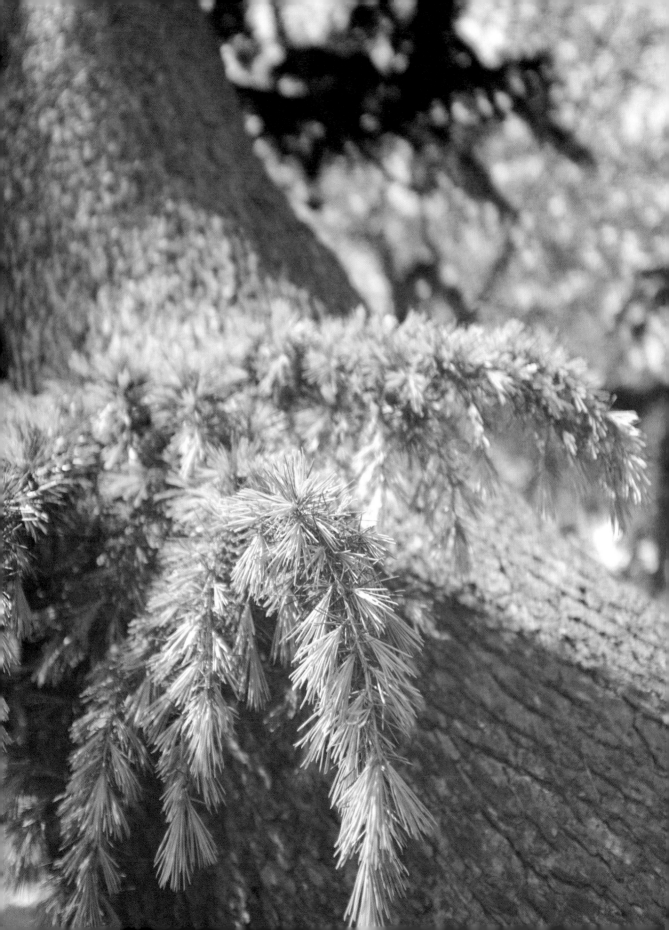

Body sweep

We often start our treelaxation with a few deep breaths and a body sweep, which means moving your attention across your body. This can take 10–15 minutes, so try to find a quiet place where you can sit or lie down comfortably and safely stay relaxed, preferably under a tree canopy. You can decide to close your eyes if you feel safe. Throughout the exercise, remember to take slow, deep, diaphragmatic breaths.

1 Move your attention to your body. Notice any sensations in the body parts that are in contact with the ground or whatever you are sitting or lying on.

2 You can then move your attention through your body. Imagine that you're shining a spotlight on the body part that you are paying attention to and simply observe any sensations that occur. Let go of the need to name or analyse them; simply allow them to come and go.

3 Notice your feet as if you are lightly touching them with your attention. Observe any sensations in the soles and tops of your feet. Then move your attention up your legs to your ankles, calves, knees, thighs and hips.

4 Move your attention to your lower abdomen, your stomach area and your chest.

5 Move your attention to your back. Observe sensations in your lower, middle and upper back. Remember, there is no need to analyse or try to change them.

6 Move your attention to your shoulders, upper arms, elbows, forearms, wrists, tops of your hands and palms of your hands. What do you notice?

7 Focus your attention on the back of your neck, the back of your head, the top of your head, your forehead, eyebrows, eyes, cheeks, nose, mouth and throat.

8 Now, observe your whole body, from the soles of your feet to the top of your head. What sensations do you notice? How do you feel? Do any body parts or areas stand out to you?

9 If you have kept your eyes closed, you can finish the exercise with a few deep, diaphragmatic breaths and gently open your eyes in your own time.

Benefits of the body sweep exercise

The body sweep exercise allows you to slow down, unwind and relax, and become more in tune with how your body feels. It is a great exercise to carry out in nature, but you can also try it at home or in your office during your lunch break; just make sure you can stay undisturbed for the whole duration. For added relaxation, you might choose to lie down. In fact, the exercise is also excellent for helping you to fall asleep, so is perfect to do before bedtime. You can find free recordings for body sweeps online.

You might notice that you feel different after a body sweep – lighter or heavier, sleepy or energized. You might even notice changes in your body – for example, you might notice a few aches appearing, or that an existing pain is no longer there. All these reactions are normal and happen due to our body swapping to the parasympathetic branch of our autonomic nervous system, which allows us to become more aware of how we truly feel.

If you can, try to honour your body's needs. The more you tune in and learn to work with your body's needs, rather than against them, the greater changes you might start seeing not only in how your body feels but also in your general mood and wellbeing.

Sensory experience

After you have observed your body, you can take a few moments to notice your senses. If it is safe and you feel comfortable, close your eyes and take a few deep breaths.

Begin by listening to the sounds closest to you (maybe your breath or the rustling of leaves on the ground), then listen to any sounds further away (perhaps the sound of the wind in the trees or birdsong) and finally move your attention as far away as you can and listen to any distant sounds (birds singing far away, the wind moving through the trees beyond those you can see or the sound of a spring at the edge of the park or forest).

You can then move your attention to your sense of touch, starting with the parts of your body where you have bare skin, like your face or hands. Notice the temperature and movement of the air on the surface of your skin. Once again, draw your attention to the parts of your body that are in contact with the ground. How do they feel?

Take a few deep breaths and open your eyes. Look into the canopy of the trees above you. You can simply observe the whole tree canopy or maybe focus on noticing colours, shapes, variations in shades of colour, textures and different sizes of leaves and branches. It can also be very therapeutic to observe the sky through the canopy of trees or notice fractals by tracing branches on a tree.

You can stay there as long as you like, simply enjoying the peaceful atmosphere. You can also continue taking in deep breaths to further induce relaxation and increase the absorption of beneficial chemicals. Notice how you feel.

Benefits of earthing

Whenever you are in nature, you can connect with it through earthing.

Earthing, also known as grounding, refers to the practice of making direct physical contact with the Earth's surface, such as having bare skin contact with the grass, sand or soil. This practice is based on the concept that the Earth's surface has a natural electric charge, and, although studies have been limited and conflicted, that connecting with it can have various health benefits.

The hypothesis is that, during earthing, mobile electrons from the Earth enter your body and act as natural antioxidants, helping to reduce inflammation in the body.[24]

There are also some studies showing that earthing can help improve mood[25] and reduce stress.[26] Other studies even suggest that earthing can help reduce pain, possibly due to its anti-inflammatory effects.[27]

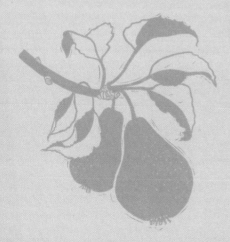

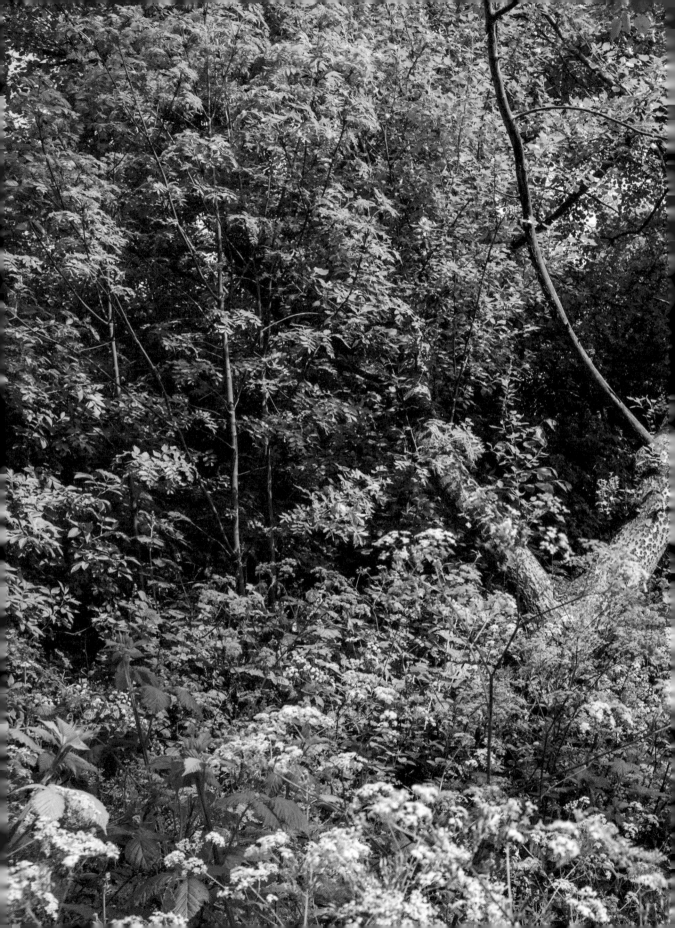

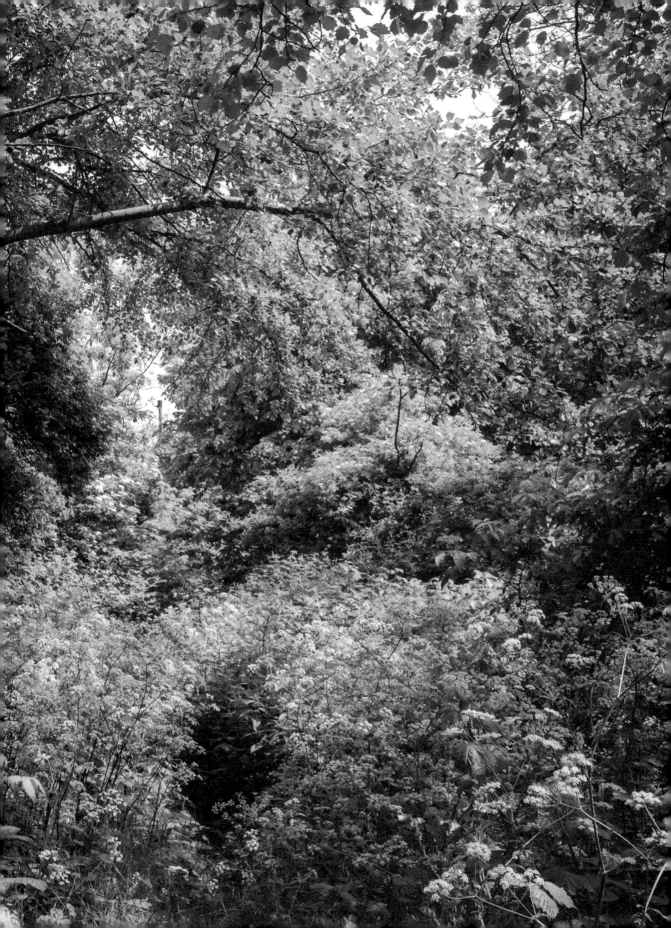

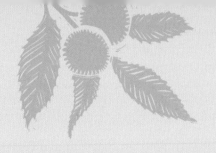

Forest bathing with children

Nature exposure has been shown to have a strong positive effect on the health and wellbeing of children. One study has found that there is a positive correlation between nature connection and improved health and life satisfaction in children,[28] while, according to Natural England, there is a lot of evidence to suggest children who spend time outside connecting with nature have better school attendance records, are more well-behaved, achieve more academically and possess stronger social skills, such as teamwork.[29]

Forest bathing is a great way to encourage kids to connect with nature in a creative and respectful way.

Depending on their age, some children might be initially sceptical about trying out forest bathing, but most seem to enjoy it a lot and often are very creative in the process, coming up with their own unique ways to explore and connect with nature.

When our baby was only a few weeks old, we started taking him out in a pram, and later in a carrier, to a nearby forest. It was truly a lifesaver, especially in the lockdown during the Covid pandemic, when we could not see our relatives and felt we were struggling with the new baby on top of work and the uncertain situation brought around by the pandemic. We found huge solace in our walks in nature – not only did our baby become calm (he was really fascinated by everything around and was eager to explore nature even from a very young age), but these walks gave us a much-needed break from all the worries and uncertainties that day-to-day life brought us. Looking back at those times, we really cherish them and are so grateful for the role that nature played in our coping as a family with a newborn.

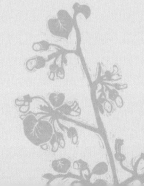

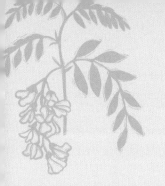
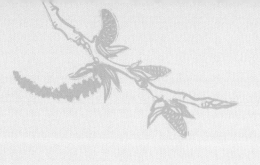
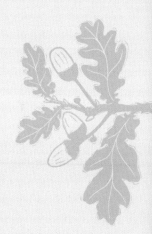

At The Forest Bathing Institute, we are lucky to be able to run forest bathing sessions for different groups, and out of all the different people we have had the privilege to work with, sessions for children are particularly enjoyable. It brings immense joy to see how many of the children are transformed simply by being in the woods and engaging with nature using their senses. It's impossible not to smile when you see the sincere joy and fascination on their faces as they show off something beautiful or unusual they have found – a piece of rare lichen, wild mushrooms, acorns or chestnuts on the ground. And when children join the sessions with their parents, it is always surprising to see how they are initially shy but then encourage and even lead their parents, showing them ways to connect with nature.

Indeed, for children, once they get over the initial shyness, connecting with nature using the senses seems very natural, and they get a lot out of it. Often, at the end of our sessions, children want to explore the forest further – they do not want to leave this magical environment.

Interestingly, we even had a very good response to our sessions among teenagers and young adults. Although some were sceptical at first, we saw them developing natural curiosity and opening up as the session went by, eager to learn more and share their experiences with others.

And while there is no one way to help children connect with nature – since children, like adults, are all beautifully different, unique individuals – there are a few tips that we can share with you to help encourage your kids to share forest bathing practice with you.

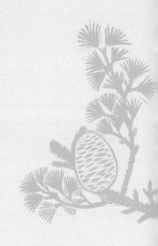

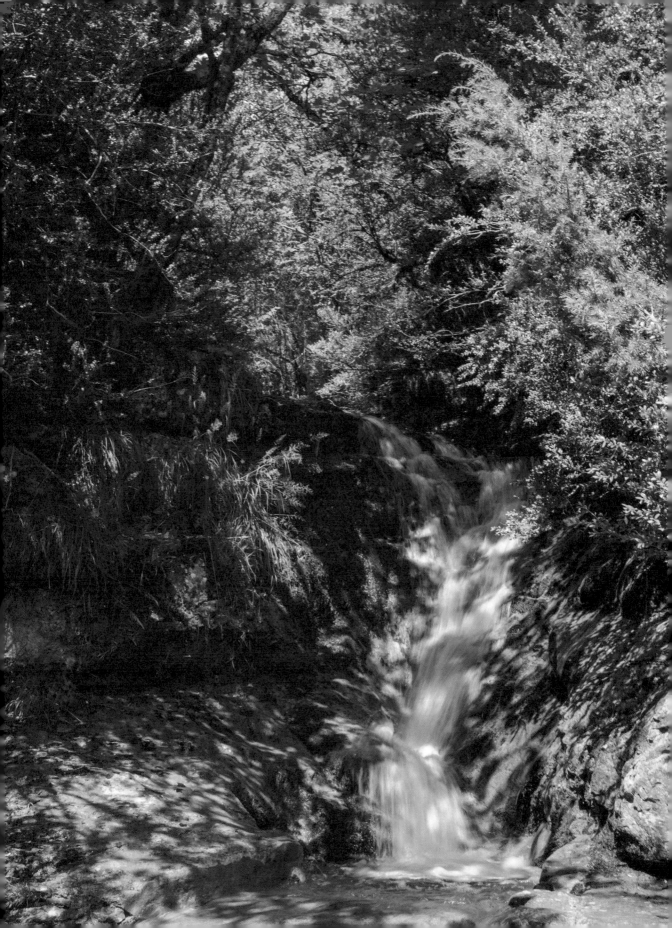

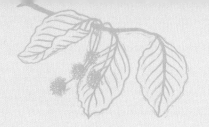

Make it fun

Rather than making forest bathing something that kids *have* to do, or something that is quite serious and formal, make a game out of it! For instance, when you are in nature, and there are lots of colours around, ask them to count how many colours they can see around them (this exercise can be part of learning for younger kids, too). Or, if you walk by an interesting tree, touch the bark and ask your kids to explore what it feels like.

Let them choose

Once you get your kids interested in forest bathing, it might be helpful to just let them be guided by their senses. Kids are often very creative, and once they get the gist of the game, they tend to roll with it. Let your kids explore nature in the way that feels most comfortable for them. For instance, you might initially ask them to listen to the sound of the birds, but they might be drawn instead to the sound of running water and try to follow it to find the stream. As long as they stay safe and do not harm nature or others, any and every way they choose to explore nature is a great way!

Give it time

If your kids are not very interested in trying out the exercises, forest bathing might not be for them, or maybe it is just not the right time. We are all individuals, and what works for one person might not work in the same way for another. Being kind, compassionate and understanding of the needs of others, as well as our own, is the key. Often, children (and also partners and other family members) get interested in what you are doing once they see positive changes in you, so as long as you take time to practise forest bathing, you might indirectly be affecting your whole family!

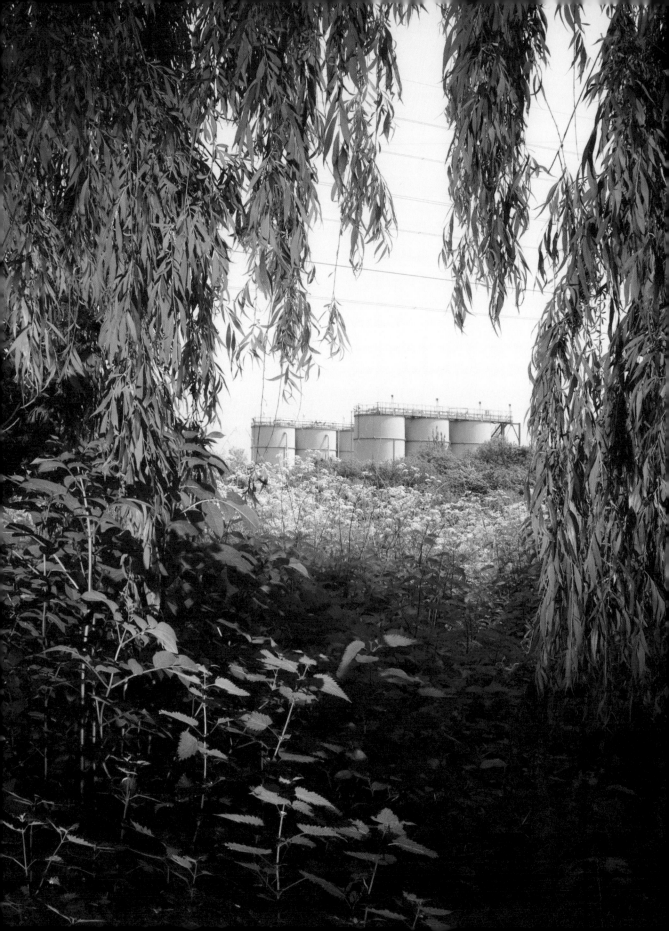

Chapter five

Bringing nature to you

You may not always be able to include nature in your day. Maybe you have limited mobility or are unable to go outside, or you might be too busy with work (we all get those days ahead of deadlines!) or perhaps your child is ill. However, there are lots of factors that contribute to the health and wellbeing effects of spending time in nature, and you can still reap some of these benefits by introducing nature indoors. Especially built natural environments and cultivated plants can provide much benefit to our health and wellbeing.

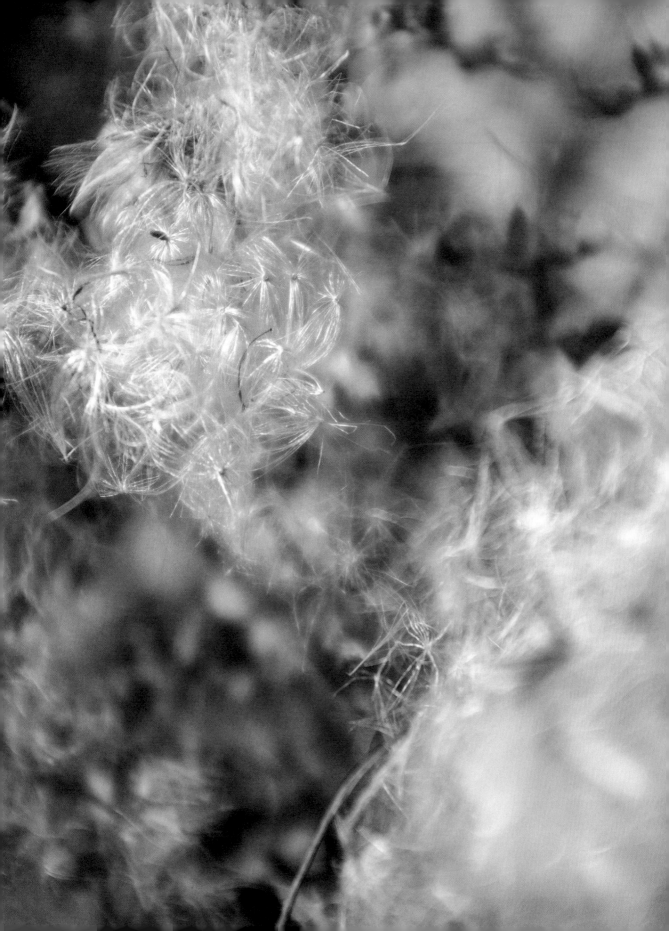

Cultivate your own garden

If you live somewhere where you have access to a garden or a patch of land that you can cultivate, you can reap many of the benefits that gardening can bring.

Gardening allows you to connect with nature on a very profound level (what better way to connect than through food?) Putting your hands into the soil can even improve your mood, due to beneficial bacteria in the soil (see page 129). On top of this, nothing beats the joyful feeling of watching a seed grow into a sapling and then into a healthy adult plant, bearing fruit that ends up on your table.

Not all of us will have the outside space or free time to garden, but you can still introduce some elements and benefits of gardening into your life by growing herbs at home. You do not need much for this – herbs can even grow on your window sill, as long as there is exposure to natural light and you keep them watered. Looking at your herbs and observing how they grow and change daily can be very rewarding, allowing you to connect with nature even on days when you are unable to go outside.

House plants
and phytoremediation

If you live somewhere where you do not have access to a garden or a patch of land where you can cultivate plants, you can still introduce nature via house plants.

House plants can help absorb and metabolize certain pollutants from the air through their leaves, roots and soil, thereby improving the overall air quality in indoor spaces. Moreover, during photosynthesis, plants take in carbon dioxide and release oxygen. This natural process helps increase oxygen levels in indoor environments, which can have a positive impact on air quality and overall wellbeing. This process is known as phytoremediation.

Some common house plants known for their air-purifying properties include spider plants, peace lilies, snake plants, pothos and rubber plants. By incorporating these plants into your indoor environment and providing them with proper care, you can help improve air quality.

Be aware that some plants absorb oxygen and release carbon dioxide at night, potentially affecting your sleep. However, low-maintenance succulents or cacti are generally considered safe in a bedroom. Be aware, too, that some people are allergic to pollen or other plant substances. If this applies to you, you can choose plants that are hypoallergenic or have low pollen counts. Finally, be careful if you have pets, as some plants (for example, peace lilies) are toxic to animals such as cats and dogs.

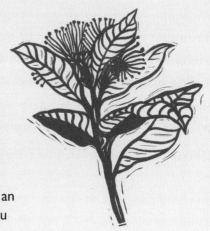

Office nature connection

You can carry out this exercise discretely at your workplace. This is an excellent exercise when you need a mental break; for example, if you are stuck on something and need a bit of inspiration or motivation.

For this exercise, you will need a plant, preferably on your desk. It is also great if this plant is within arm's reach and comfortable to touch (cacti are not ideal!)

1 Focus your attention on the plant. Slowly observe its shape by following its edges with your eyes, from the base up to the top on one side of the plant, and down the other side. If you feel like it, you can trace each leaf's shape with your eyes as well. As you do this exercise, take slow deep breaths in and out through your nose.

2 If you have time, you can also spend a few moments noticing different colours and shades of a colour on a plant. How do the shades of the colour change? Do you notice any difference in the intensity of the colour from the previous time you looked at the plant?

3 If you have a few more minutes to spare, you can gently touch the plant. Feel the difference in the texture between the leaves, the stem, flowers and other parts of the plant. Experiment using different fingers to slowly run your fingertips over the surface of the plant. How does it feel?

4 Take a few more deep breaths before you restart your work. You may notice that you feel more focused, clear-minded and even rejuvenated – like you have had a refreshing mini-break.

Through a window

If you are unable to use a space outside or to introduce house plants where you live, there are other ways to bring nature into your day-to-day life.

If you are lucky to live or work somewhere surrounded by nature, where you can see trees, grass and other greenery outside your window, you can anchor your attention on these natural elements and take time to explore them, similarly to how you would a house plant (although, of course, you will probably be unable to touch them when you are indoors).

You can also notice movement. This can be especially rewarding on a windy day, when you observe the tops of the trees swaying in the wind. Once you come back from this relaxing activity, you might find that your attention and focus have sharpened, and you have a new sense of rejuvenation and energy to tackle tasks at hand – whether it is sorting out bills at home or answering emails at work.

Once you come back from this relaxing activity, you might find that your attention and focus have sharpened, and you have a new sense of rejuvenation and energy

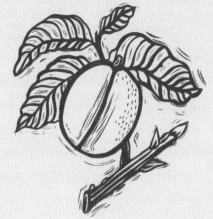

Attention Restoration Theory

Attention Restoration Theory (ART) is a psychological concept that suggests exposure to natural environments can help restore cognitive resources and improve attention and focus. Developed by psychologists Rachel and Stephen Kaplan in the 1980s, ART posits that spending time in nature can have restorative effects on mental fatigue and attentional capacities, leading to improved cognitive performance and wellbeing.[30]

ART distinguishes between two types of attention: directed attention, which is required for tasks that demand focus and concentration; and involuntary attention, which is more effortless and occurs when we are in natural settings.

Directed attention can become fatigued with prolonged use, leading to decreased cognitive performance, increased stress and mental exhaustion. This fatigue can be alleviated by spending time in natural environments, which promote involuntary attention.

Natural settings, characterized by elements such as greenery, water and natural sounds, are considered restorative environments that facilitate psychological restoration and replenishment of cognitive resources. Nature provides what the Kaplans termed 'soft fascination', which captures our attention in a gentle, effortless way, allowing directed attention to rest and recover.

While direct exposure to nature might have the strongest effect, indirect exposure, such as looking at nature through a window or listening to natural sounds, can also help alleviate the symptoms of fatigue, restore attention and improve cognitive performance.

Nature sights and sounds

It is interesting that nature has such a powerful effect on our psychology that even something as simple as introducing nature imagery or natural sounds into our day-to-day life can have a strong positive effect on our mood and even behaviour.

Natural imagery seems to have a profound calming effect on our minds. For instance, one study followed inmates in solitary confinement in an Oregon prison for a year, and found that those who viewed nature videos several times a week committed 26 per cent fewer violent infractions than their peers.[31]

Similarly, nature sounds can also have a profound effect on how relaxed we feel. In our 2019 study with the University of Derby, we found that one of the settings in which participants were most relaxed during forest bathing was when listening to the sound of moving water.

Try printing nature pictures from the internet, which you can find royalty-free on some websites, invest in pleasing nature landscape paintings or prints, or even come back to the nature photography in this book! You can also change the screensavers on your computer and your phone to a pleasing natural landscape.

There are also a great variety of natural sounds you can listen to online and download for free. Choose natural sounds that are most appealing to you. The sounds of birds, running water, wind or rain are some top hits!

Listen to natural sounds whenever you have an opportunity to do so – on your commute to and from work, when you are doing house chores, working or simply winding down for the day. For a deeper relaxation experience, sit with your eyes closed where you will not be disturbed, play the recording (headphones might be best for this) and relax for a couple of minutes. This could also be a great idea for a mini-break at work, and can even help you fall asleep at night.

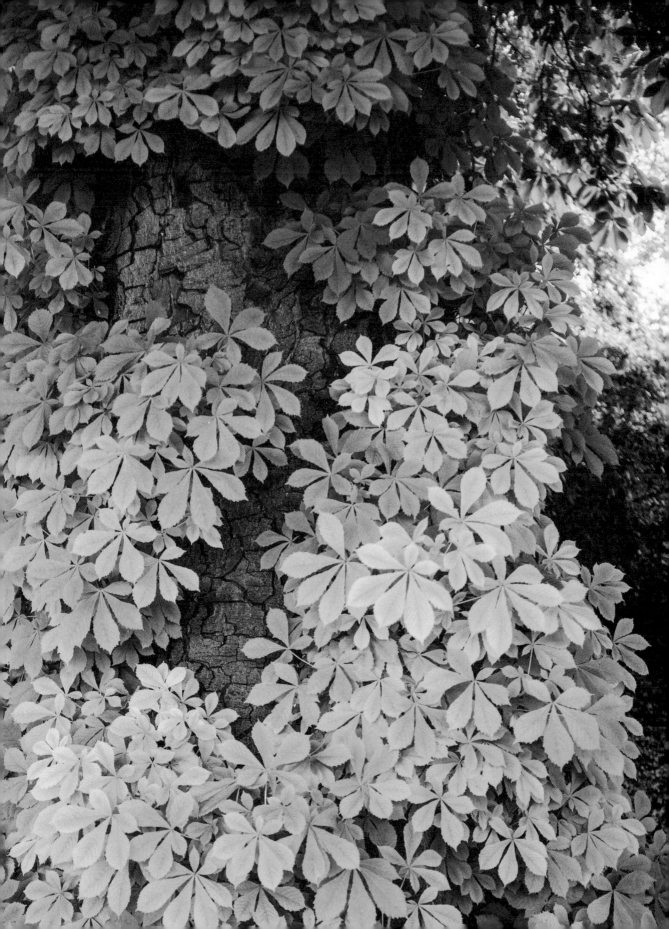

The scents of nature

As we have already mentioned, research by Professor Li into the properties of phytoncides (see page 59) has revealed that these contribute up to 50 per cent of the health-giving benefits of spending time within a woodland or forest environment. And, fortunately, phytoncides are not only found in forests.

Some examples of plants that give off phytoncides that can be found outside forests are cedar, garlic, locust, oak, onion, pine and tea tree, among others. As phytoncides are released by plants as a reaction to an injury or disease, you will only receive the benefits from living plants. However, you can also get phytoncide exposure with the usage of essential oils from the plants listed above.

Our connection to nature will be different for each of us but we can always strengthen it by reinforcing it on a daily basis

Too busy by half

Here are some ideas to help incorporate nature connection into your day-to-day life if you can't easily get out regularly into nature:

- **Walking your children to school:** You can make something as mundane as a walk to and from school an opportunity for you and your children to connect with nature. On the walk, dedicate a few minutes to walking in silence and soaking up the nature around you, and/or use some of the family-friendly forest bathing activities from Chapter 4.
- **Cycling to/from work:** Forest bathing is obviously not advisable when cycling and/or driving a car, as you need to focus on the road (though you can do it if you are in a passenger seat). But if you cycle to and from work, why not dedicate the last 10 –15 minutes of your journey to observing nature around you while walking alongside your bicycle?
- **Running in nature:** Going for a run in nature can be very rewarding. Not only do we get to immerse ourselves in nature, but the increased blood circulation can boost our oxygen intake, and we might be able to reap some other benefits from exercise too. However, what is important to remember about forest bathing practice is that it is a slow-paced practice. And while you might be immersed in nature while running, it would be very hard to say that you are forest bathing. We give the same advice regarding running as we do for cycling. Instead of trying to combine the two, why not dedicate some of the time to running and the rest to forest bathing? You will find that this approach is often more manageable and enjoyable, as you can then fully immerse yourself into each of the activities without unnecessary complications or interruptions.
- **Family picnic:** Perhaps not possible every day, but it would be great to go out for a picnic whenever you can. Dedicate at least 20 minutes of the picnic to exploring nature alone in silence, keeping in sight of each other if you have young children. Or engage your family with some of our family-friendly forest bathing activities (see Chapter 4).

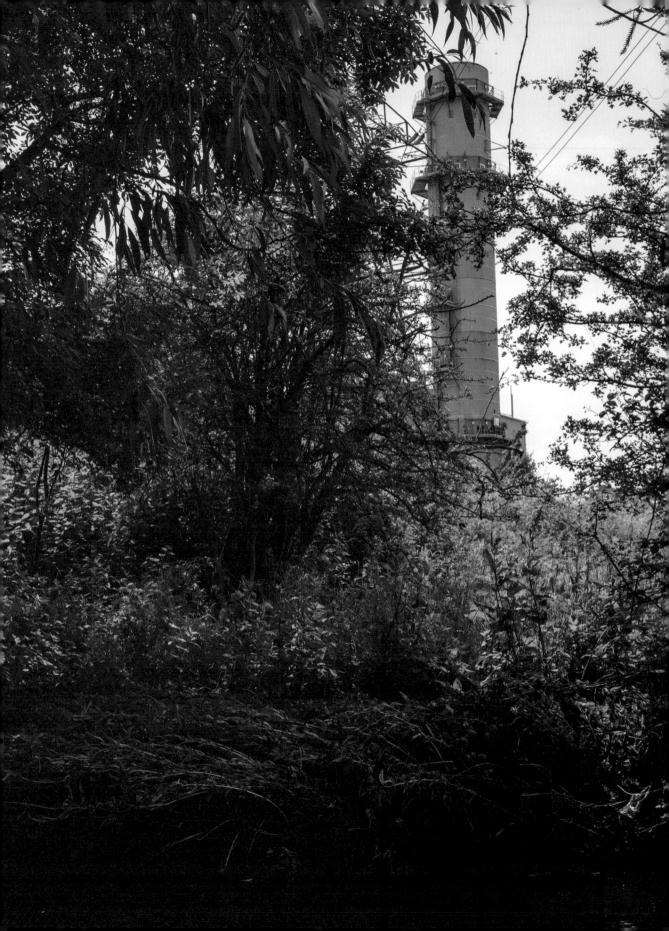

Connection and gratitude

Most of us associate nature with something that we can connect with when going outside to a park, a nature reserve or a forest. But in reality, it plays a crucial part in our day-to-day life whether we go outside or not, and this is because we are part of it. It is in the air we breathe, the food we eat and the water we drink, the light we perceive … If you think about it, all our essential life-sustaining activities of the day revolve around nature – we simply forget about it.

Next time you enjoy a meal or become mindful of your breath, remember that you are always connected to nature with every breath you take. In that moment, it might help to feel gratitude towards nature and what it brings you. Alternatively, you can simply sit with this feeling of connection, being part of something bigger.

Whether you go outside into nature or enjoy nature indoors, any daily activity you do can link to nature, as long as you keep the intention. For you are part of nature – something worth contemplating.

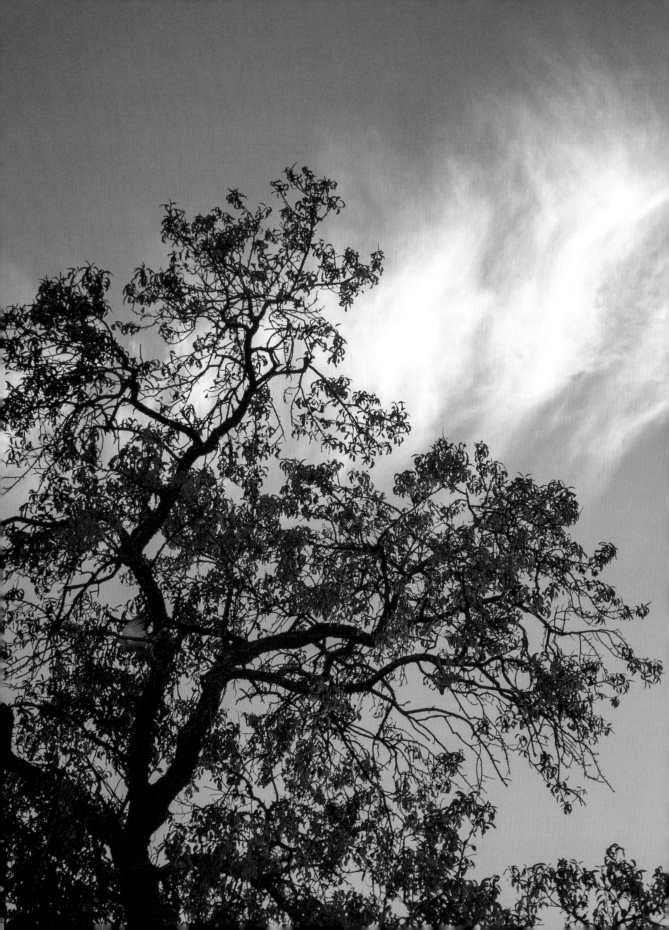

Chapter six

Building a forest bathing habit

Once we set an intention, we might be faced with a few challenges on our way to achieving our goal. Some of the common reasons why people find it challenging to stick to new resolutions are a lack of motivation or commitment, unrealistic goals, lack of accountability, fear of failure and not having a clear plan, as well as circumstances outside of our control.

Many of us might have been caught up in a cycle of making promises around the new year. The idea of a 'new me', a better, healthier version of oneself, seems so enticing!

Resolutions have been known for centuries in different ancient traditions, commencing with the Vedic tradition of 'sankalpa', a Sanskit word that refers to making vows and intentions. Making resolutions can be very helpful to give our actions a direction and to set up goals.

There are many reasons why we might be starting a new habit, and while a number of these can be incredibly helpful in keeping us motivated, sometimes the reasons might not be strong enough to keep our motivation going. For instance, think of the last time you tried an activity just because your friends were recommending it, or because it was the hottest trend of the month. If you did not have additional good reasons to try the activity – for example, concern for your health and wellbeing, or an interest or curiosity in the subject – you might have found that the initial thrill of trying something new soon wore off.

Equally, you might have all the right reasons for taking up a new practice, but unless you have a clear plan on how to move forwards with this, you may find yourself struggling to keep it up.

Doubt and fear of failure can cause us to practise less, or even to stop altogether.

Furthermore, we should not forget that alongside all the possible difficulties that we may face in setting up a habit, we might also experience external circumstances that make it more challenging to continue our practice. An urgent deadline at work, the sickness of a child, unplanned repairs at home, challenges in relationships – all these factors (and many others) can, sadly, switch our focus from our wellbeing to the emergencies we have to deal with there and then.

While addressing all these challenges might be beyond the scope of this book, we hope that some of the tips in this chapter will help motivate you to continue your forest bathing practice and assist in creating a wonderful, health-boosting, sustainable habit that you can enjoy for years, if not decades, to come.

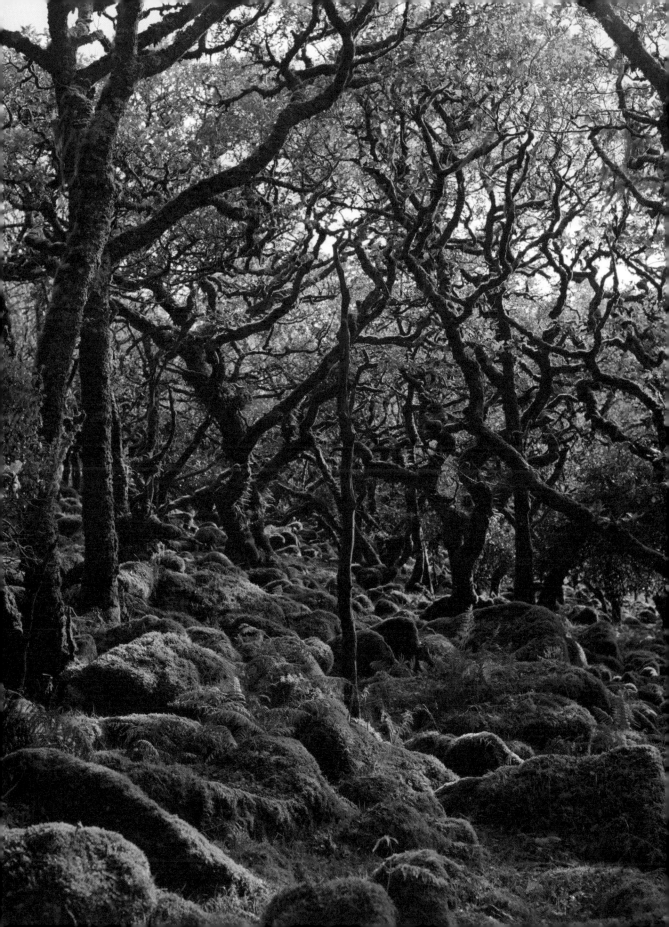

Find your 'why'

With the fast pace of life that many of us experience, even the thought of introducing a new habit might be challenging.

The fact is, our lives tend to be quite busy. And unless we make the effort to slow things down and make conscious decisions, we are likely to end up trying everything and anything. The result can often be frustration for not being able to achieve a desired goal, which can lead to simply giving up or forgetting about our intentions altogether.

Try to remember the last time you found something you really liked – it could be a new hobby or health craze. How did it make you feel? What made you want to try this activity? Finding your reason 'why' can be a strong ally in helping you keep your practice long term.

When you feel your motivation start to flag, remind yourself why you are pursuing this goal in the first place: ask yourself why forest bathing is important to you.

Some of the reasons people try forest bathing are to spend more time in nature, boost health and wellbeing, reduce stress, improve creativity, increase connection with nature, care for nature and leave a positive impact – and there are many others!

From the above list, you can choose the reasons that resonate the most with you, or you can create your own list of motivations for practising forest bathing.

Every time you struggle to keep to your practice, you can review your list of motivating factors and see if these still resonate with you. If not, you might need to review your list and see if you can find different reasons that will motivate you more effectively to continue, or come back to the list in a week or two, once you have a clearer picture in your mind of why you want to forest bathe, to see if you still find your list of reasons for practising forest bathing inspiring.

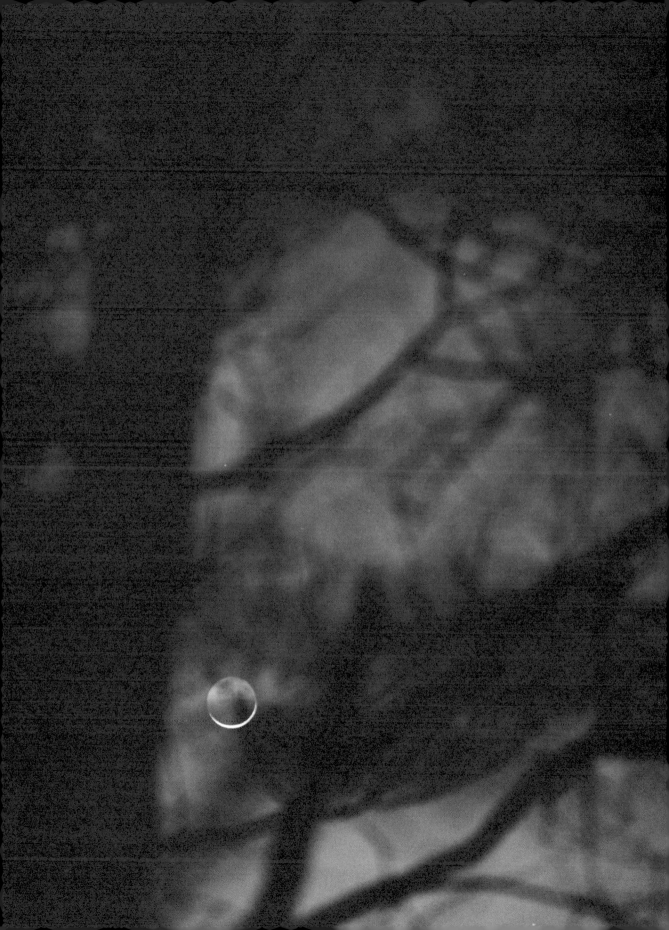

Find the time

Regularity is often key to creating a habit. A 2009 study on habit creation followed people who took up a new daily activity – eating a piece of fruit with lunch or running for 15 minutes before dinner – and found that it took an average of 66 days (ranging between 18 days and 254 days) for these activities to become automatic habits. According to Phillippa Lally, one of the authors of the study, daily repetition was the biggest factor influencing whether a behaviour would become part of an automatic daily routine.[32]

This study demonstrates that, firstly, the time it takes for a habit to form will vary from person to person – some might take months to create a habit, while others might take weeks. Second, regularity and daily uninterrupted repetition are some of the most reliable factors in forming a habit. In other words, consistency is key.

Bearing in mind these findings, we recommend that you set aside at least 20 minutes a day to spend in nature.

You might want to choose a tree-lined street to walk along on your way to work or school in the morning, rather than taking a car or a bus, or you could get off the bus a few stops before your destination to enjoy a mindful stroll through a park on your way to work (or park your car a few blocks away and walk).

You can also try going out into nature during your lunch breaks. This is something I (Olga) did every day when I was living in central London back in 2014, at the beginning of my nature connection journey. I was lucky with the location of my office and could enjoy the beautiful grounds of St Paul's Cathedral, which had majestic old trees, as well as lovely cosy benches to sit on and enjoy my lunch while I watched squirrels playing in the trees or felt the wind on my skin.

Another favourite of mine is an early morning walk (in a safe area). I love waking up just before sunrise and going out for a walk in nature. I can't describe to you the peace and joy I get out of this habit!

It feels like I am in a different world, somewhere far away from the hustle and bustle of everyday life, witnessing the world awaken. Depending on the weather and where you are, you might also be treated to a spectacular sunrise. For me, this is the most beautiful natural phenomenon that we can observe every day.

I also really like evening walks in nature after work. If you find yourself rushing in the morning and think you will find it difficult to relax and slow down enough to enjoy time in nature at the start of the day, evening walks might be a solution. (Although, it is worth noting that if you were to do a morning walk on a daily basis, you might find it becomes easier to relax, even during busy mornings.) It is very satisfying to watch the world slow down, listen to the evening sounds of owls hooting, observe the birds settling in for the night, perhaps even watch a beautiful sunset!

However, one factor to consider if you opt for evening walks is the daylight – you might be able to do evening walks after work in spring, summer and autumn, but in winter, when the sun sets earlier, it may be better to go for a lunchtime or morning walk instead. Once you have successfully implemented a daily habit of forest bathing, you can move up the Nature Pyramid (see pages 40–1) and begin to introduce longer, monthly immersions in wilder environments and annual nature breaks. The critical point here is not to get overwhelmed – if you feel you are still struggling with daily forest bathing, it might be worth waiting to introduce longer immersions. Quality is more important than quantity.

Habits

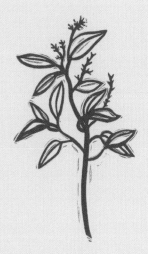

A habit is a routine behaviour or action that is regularly repeated and tends to occur subconsciously. Habits are often ingrained through repetition and can be either positive or negative. Positive habits contribute to personal growth, wellbeing and productivity, while negative habits can hinder progress or have adverse effects on one's life. Developing good habits and breaking bad ones can have a significant impact on overall health, happiness and success.

Know yourself

While regularity is one of the main factors in determining the success of establishing a habit, it is important to remember that we are all individuals. What takes someone a few months can take another person a few weeks or even days.

One of the factors predetermining the success and speed of implementing a new habit is neuroplasticity – the brain's ability to adapt and change by forming new pathways and connections between neurons. Neuroplasticity plays a crucial role in cognitive functions, including learning, memory and recovery from brain injuries. Neuroplasticity is a fabulous ability, and great news for people of all ages. The science of neuroplasticity tells us that we are capable of positive change whatever age we are, and our brain will work with us to support new, healthy habits. Thus we can work with neuroplasticity to help ourselves.

Neuroplasticity is one of the factors that can determine how fast and how successful we will be at implementing a new habit, like forest bathing. Various factors can influence one's neuroplasticity, such as age, environment, experience and learning, genetics, physical exercise, and physical and mental health. But, interestingly, one thing that has been shown to help improve our neuroplasticity is mindfulness.[33] As mindfulness involves focusing attention on the present moment, this, in turn, can bring about structural changes in the brain that may be linked to enhanced neuroplasticity.

Learning a new practice, like forest bathing, can be challenging at first, but the good news is that while we are learning this practice, we might be helping develop neuroplasticity in our brain, which can have its own benefits.

We all have different needs, lifestyles and obligations, such as work and family, as well as physical health and wellbeing needs; what might be easy for one person to implement might not necessarily be so easy for another. On top of this, while time in nature can be beneficial for all, we are always advocating for a balanced approach to life. It is OK if you do not have time to go into nature for one or two days – you might need to prioritize your work and other responsibilities, which is absolutely fine and very healthy.

Furthermore, it is great if you can think of forest bathing as a positive addition to your life, enhancing health and wellbeing, rather than yet another chore you are obliged to do.

Balancing the needs of your busy life and the regularity of your forest bathing practice might be quite challenging at first, but over time, as you become more used to the routine and what forest bathing involves, you may find that maintaining your practice becomes easier and does not require as much energy and commitment. Indeed, you might find that forest bathing can simultaneously increase your energy levels while reducing your stress levels, which can lead to better decision-making, prioritizing and planning skills. This, in turn, can allow you to review your current lifestyle and make changes if needed – sometimes even allowing space and time for other activities that can be helpful to your health and wellbeing. What an amazing knock-on effect!

Coming to forest bathing with an attitude of helping yourself, rather than making yourself do something you do not enjoy, can bring more benefits, as it will allow your body to relax deeper and soak up the benefits that forests can provide

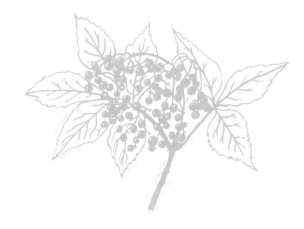

Find your community

Adjusting our regular routine to allow more time for a new practice is something that all of us might need to do by ourselves. But something that can really help us on our journey is support from our family and friends.

Remember the last time you took on a new habit or hobby? What were the reactions from your family or friends? Did you notice a difference in your motivation levels if your loved ones supported you with your pursuit?

When you start forest bathing, you might want to inform your family and friends, especially if you might need their motivational support or even practical help with work or errands (for example, you might want to ask your partner to look after the children while you are out catching your daily dose of nature).

Support from family and friends can be very useful when you need a boost to your motivation, someone to share your experience with or someone who can help you practically.

Of course, all situations are different, and we appreciate that it might not always be possible to get support from your friends and family. In this case, compassion and empathy towards yourself might be your best tools. Forest bathing might not be for everyone, but if you feel this practice can be beneficial to you, it could be helpful to remind yourself of the reasons why you started the practice in the first place. It can also be a great idea to connect with like-minded forest bathers whom you can meet during forest bathing events (you can find events on our website **www.tfb.institute**).

Connect with other readers!

We have dedicated a Facebook page for the readers of this book who would like to support each other on their forest bathing journey. You can join for free and see whom you can connect with in your area. You can find more information about it on our website: **www.tfb.institute**

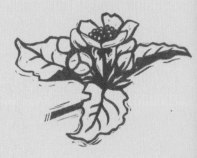

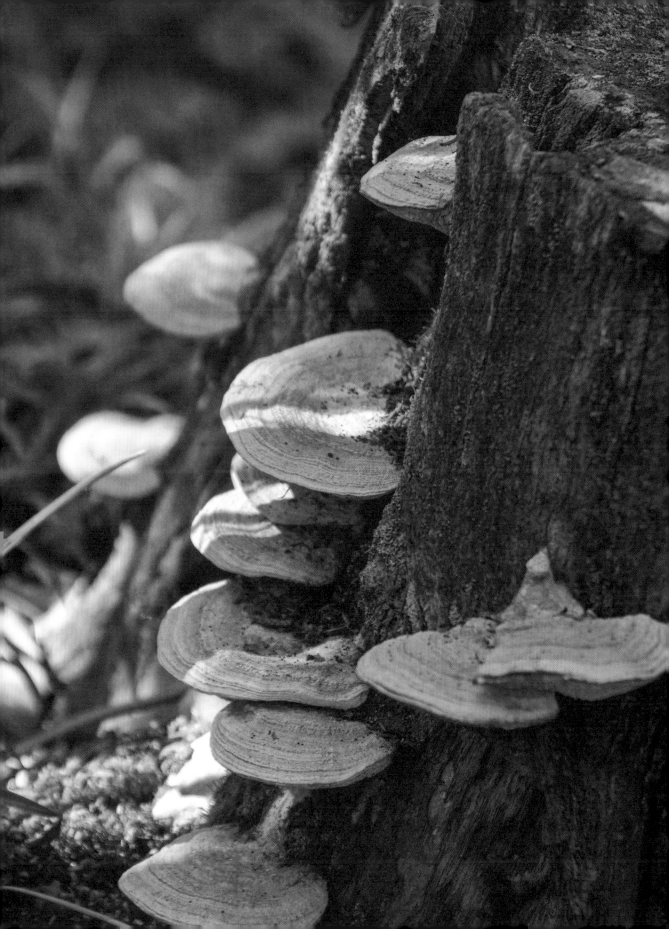

Be patient

For many people it takes time for the benefits of forest bathing – such as improved sleep, reduced stress and anxiety, and improved mood – to make themselves known. While some may see benefits even after just one walk in nature (in fact, from our experience, those who have less nature contact in their everyday life tend to see the most benefit), others might not notice any changes for weeks or months.

It is important to understand that any change takes time. Just as it takes time for our minds to adjust to the introduction of a new routine, similarly it can take time for our bodies to register the changes and show the benefits of forest bathing. It's also important to note that results might be different for everyone and may not always be what you expect them to be.

For instance, a common reaction after our forest bathing sessions is an increased sense of tiredness. Contrary to some peoples' belief, nature does not induce tiredness. Rather, it allows our nervous system to slow down so that we can notice how we truly feel. If we have been busy and not resting properly, once our bodies slow down and we are able to see how we really feel, we might start noticing feeling tired, which usually is proportionate to how much rest we need – the more you have been neglecting your rest, the more tired you might feel.

The upside of feeling tired after a forest bathing session is that our participants often report a sounder, deeper sleep. Since our bodies are more in tune with how we feel, our physiological needs are much clearer and we can notice them more easily. This can also be translated as our bodies coming into balance or to their natural state of seeking homeostasis. In this state, we are more likely to notice how we truly feel and what our bodies need – whether it is rest, food, time in nature or something else.

If you start noticing undesirable reactions in your body, such as feeling tired when you have a very busy day ahead, try to just see these reactions as your body's messages to you. If you are feeling tired, your body is sending a message that you need to slow down and rest. This does not mean that you necessarily have to react instantly once you experience these reactions (although if you are tired and can rest, your body will definitely appreciate it!) But taking this information on board and adjusting your day or maybe even your lifestyle over time might be a crucial step in building a healthy relationship between your body and mind.

Profound changes can take a while, especially if we require big changes in our way of living or how we treat ourselves. But we and thousands of other people who have been lucky enough to connect with nature and tune more into how we truly feel, reap big benefits. We tend to become much happier and healthier. We have more energy and get more enjoyment out of life, which in turn can also boost our creativity and productivity. There is never a loss when we stay connected with our true nature – even though it might seem so at the start! Trust the process and your gut. Nature will be a big help with this.

A good cry

Cortisol is a stress hormone that is present in the bloodstream and can be transported to various bodily fluids, including tears. When cortisol levels increase in response to stress, some of it may be excreted through tears as a way for the body to regulate stress levels. Tears can be a sign of release and also indicate that we have been suppressing how we truly feel.

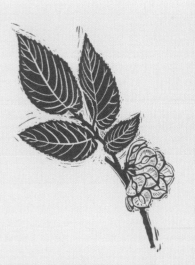

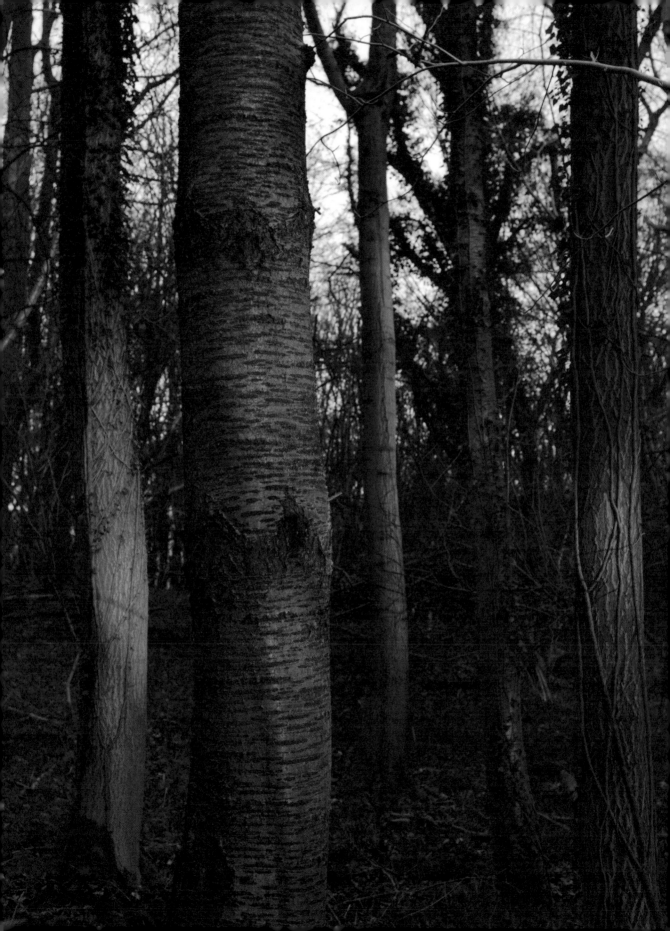

Write it out

Often, we find it challenging to observe daily changes taking place. Can you remember the last time you looked back on something and wondered where the time had gone? As you become more mindful and aware, you may start noticing changes around you in nature, as well as changes in your relatives and loved ones. Over time, it might also become easier to observe yourself as you change; you may notice all the slight changes that take place daily, as well as bigger changes happening over time.

As we build up our mindful awareness through the practice of forest bathing, it might be helpful to keep a diary. This does not have to be anything elaborate – you can even use something you already have, like an old notebook or planner, or type your daily observations on your computer or even in the notes section on your phone.

Everyone's observations will be different from day to day, but questions you might ask yourself are:

- Did I go into nature today?
- Where did I go?
- What did I notice?
- How did I feel? (You can include observations on your physical body and your emotional wellbeing.)
- Did I notice any changes on the day?

If you are more inclined to write stories, you can describe your day as a story. You can write as little or as much as you like, but if you can, try to stay consistent with your journaling practice.

Occasionally, for example once a month, you may want to review your notes to see if there are any changes, patterns or anything else that stands out to you. You might be surprised to notice changes or gain insights from your journaling that you may not have picked up on otherwise.

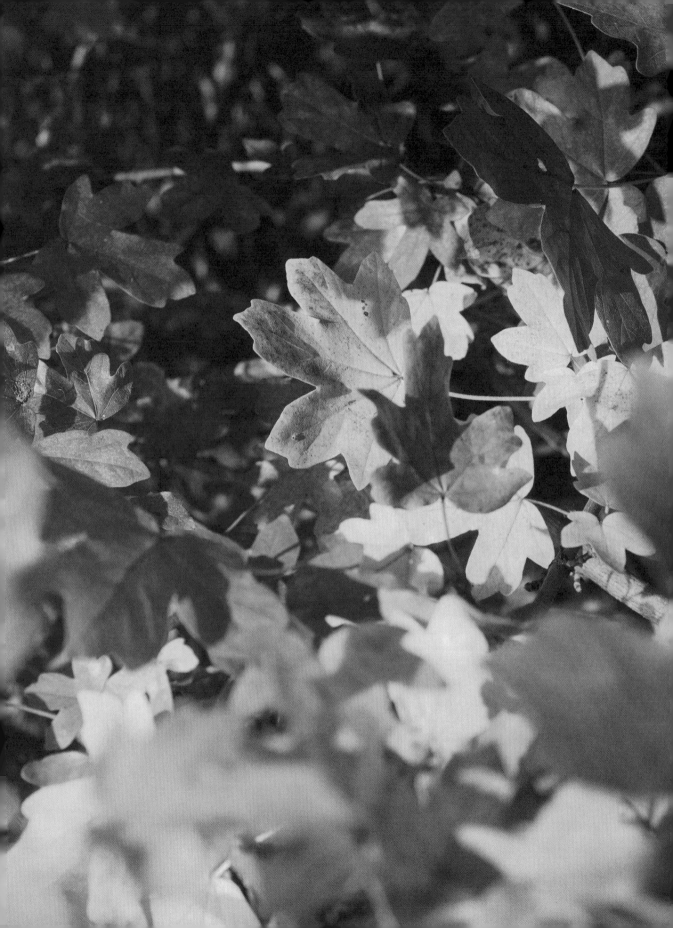

Chapter seven

How forest bathing can help the planet

If we look at our planet, we can see that it is currently facing many challenges. According to the World Wildlife Fund's *Living Planet Report 2024*, over the last half century wildlife populations have decreased by 73 per cent, with Central and South America experiencing particular decline.[34] The world has lost one-third of its forests since the end of the last ice age 10,000 years ago,[35] and half of this loss occurred in the last century alone.[36]

With its iconic English gardens, beautiful BBC wildlife documentaries and a culture of nature walks that dates back centuries, the UK is often considered to be a nation of nature lovers, yet, sadly, it is already one of the most nature-depleted areas in the world. Species have declined and one in six are now threatened with extinction,[37] plus precious woodland habitats are being lost or left to ruin.[38]

On top of this, in recent years we have experienced a drastic increase in natural disasters, including droughts, floods and wildfires. The flood and drought disasters recorded in the ten worst-hit countries have increased dramatically; for example, Somalia experienced 223 disasters in 2023, compared to just two in 2013. The Philippines, Brazil and Malaysia, among other countries, have seen a similar sharp rise in floods and droughts.[39]

And while the causes of these disasters are multiple and complex, human behaviour in the last century has been a major contributing factor to the declining health and wellbeing of our planet.

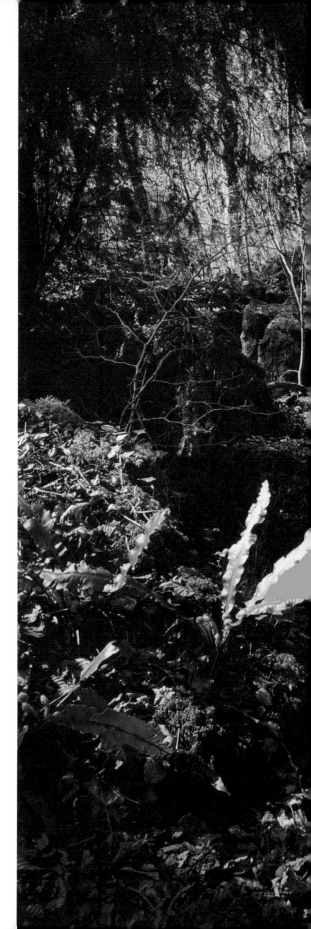

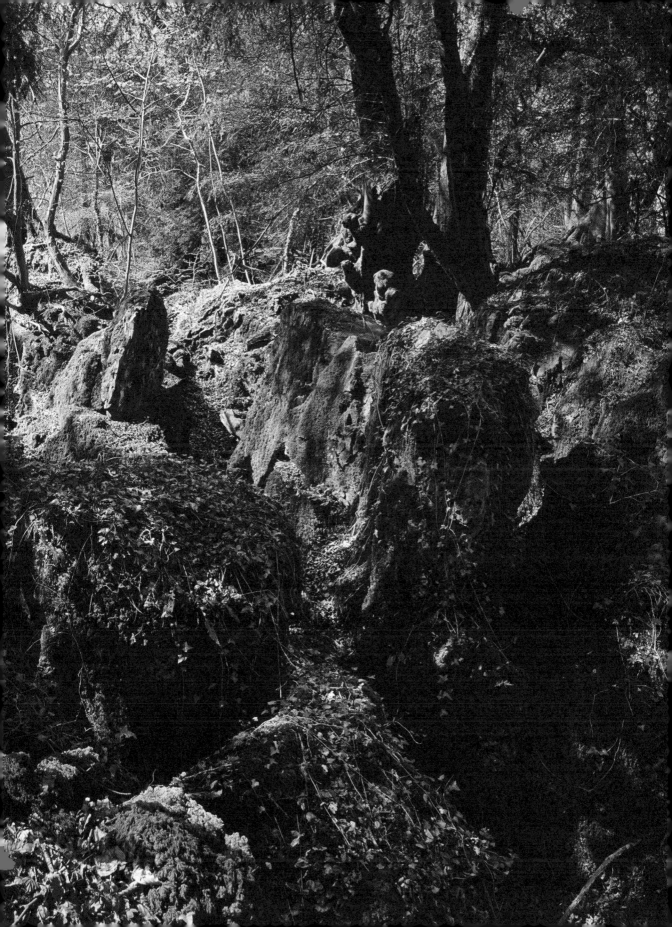

Pro-environmental behaviours

Unfortunately, there is no one magical solution to these problems. Instead, a holistic approach is required. While the direction our governments choose to take in the upcoming years will, no doubt, have a big impact on the existing situation, our individual actions and choices can also play a huge role.

When we talk about pro-environmental behaviours, some of us might think of peaceful protesting or political actions. While these have a vital role to play, it is often in the day-to-day little things that we can see the most drastic changes over time. And we are not only talking about classical pro-environmental behaviours here, but also our attitudes.

Imagine how our world would look if most of us opted to walk or cycle to work or school, if it was possible, instead of taking short commutes by car? If we took time to repair our old items, instead of buying new ones?

If we let a corner of our garden go wild and had the privilege of observing rare species appear right on our doorstep? If we went for a walk in the woods every month and took time to take care of ourselves and enjoy the beauty of the natural world?

A meta-analysis of some systematic reviews published in the *Journal of Environmental Psychology* has demonstrated the link and significant causal effect between nature connectedness – which can be described as the strength of one's personal relationship with nature (rather than simply being in or visiting nature) – and pro-environmental behaviours (PEBs).[40] Their conclusion was that nature connection is a promising method for promoting pro-environmental behaviours in individuals. In addition, there are a few systematic reviews showing the link between nature connectedness and human wellbeing.[41]

Becoming a part of nature

In forest bathing, we actively connect with nature using mindful awareness through our senses. Hence, forest bathing is a wellbeing-inducing practice aimed at creating and strengthening one's connection with nature.

Often, when we connect with nature, we tend to see more value and beauty in it, and so appreciate it more. When I (Olga) first reconnected with nature after years of living in central London and rarely spending time in nature, I suddenly felt that I was part of the natural world. Nature was no longer something 'out there', something you go into simply for recreation or while exercising. It shone in a completely different light, not only forever changing my relationship with nature but also my attitudes and behaviours towards it, alongside how I saw myself in relation to the natural world. Since then, without even noticing it, my life has changed drastically. These days, I can no longer see myself as separate from nature, and, unsurprisingly, anything that concerns nature now concerns me.

When I first reconnected with nature after years of living in central London and rarely spending time in nature, I suddenly felt that I was part of the natural world

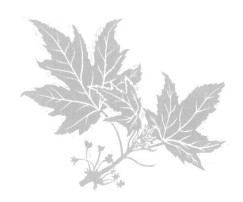

While in the past, floods, droughts and loss of species seemed like issues 'out there' – things that I could not relate to, even if I wanted to – now it feels like I am sharing these problems with nature. Unsurprisingly, this drastic change in my attitudes towards issues in the natural world has led to a drastic change in my behaviours: what and how I consume, how I travel, ways I choose to spend my time, priorities I have, life lessons I teach our four-year-old. My life has changed its perspective. While in the past I used to see myself as a small bubble floating in a big world, I now see the whole world as my bubble – a bubble I highly cherish and have a strong need to take care of.

Since I started to see myself as part of the natural world, I have also started seeing other people as part of it – no matter how different we are, we are all part of the natural world. This approach has helped me develop humility and also a deep sense of compassion towards myself and others.

Our journeys to nature connection are all unique. As you continue exploring nature, and connecting with it, you might see that your behaviours and attitudes change, and these changes will be unique to you and your particular circumstances and needs. We encourage you to have patience and observe these changes with curiosity and open-mindedness – we all have different paths to take, and your path can be a longer one and look different to another's path. Simply observing any changes that occur within you can shed light not only onto the natural world and your connection with it, but also onto your own nature.

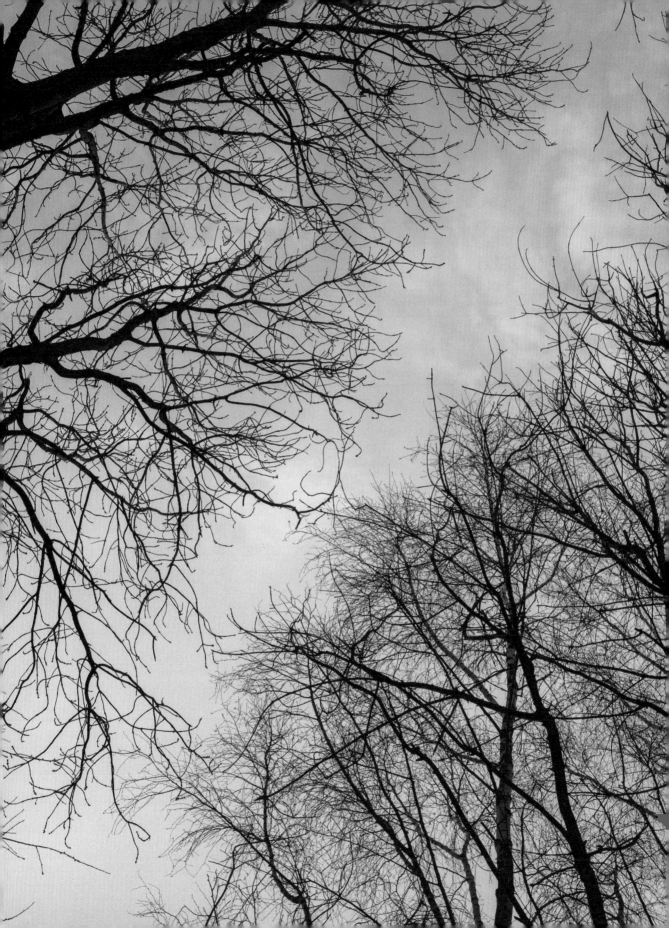

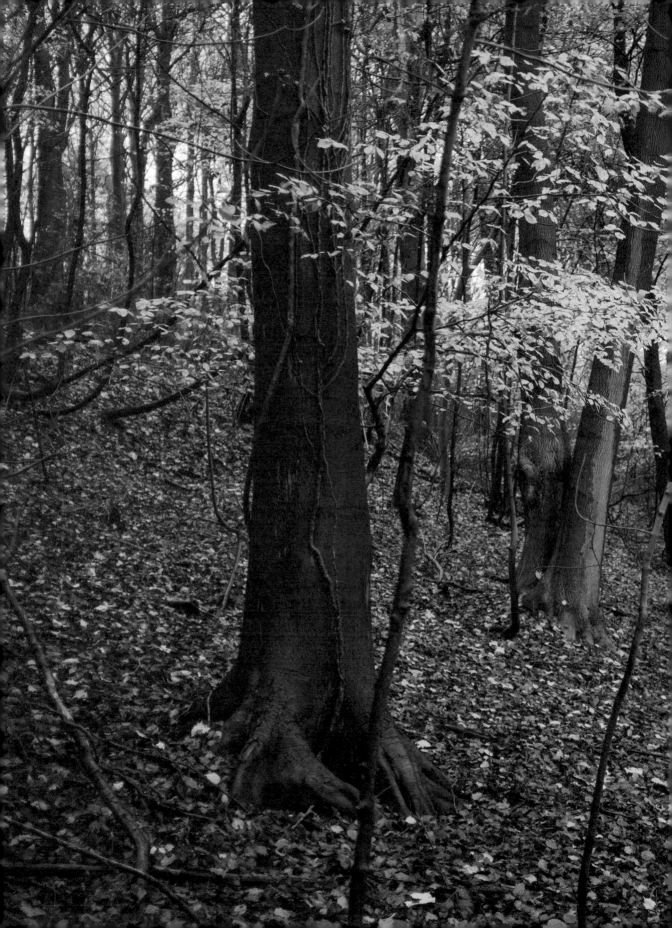

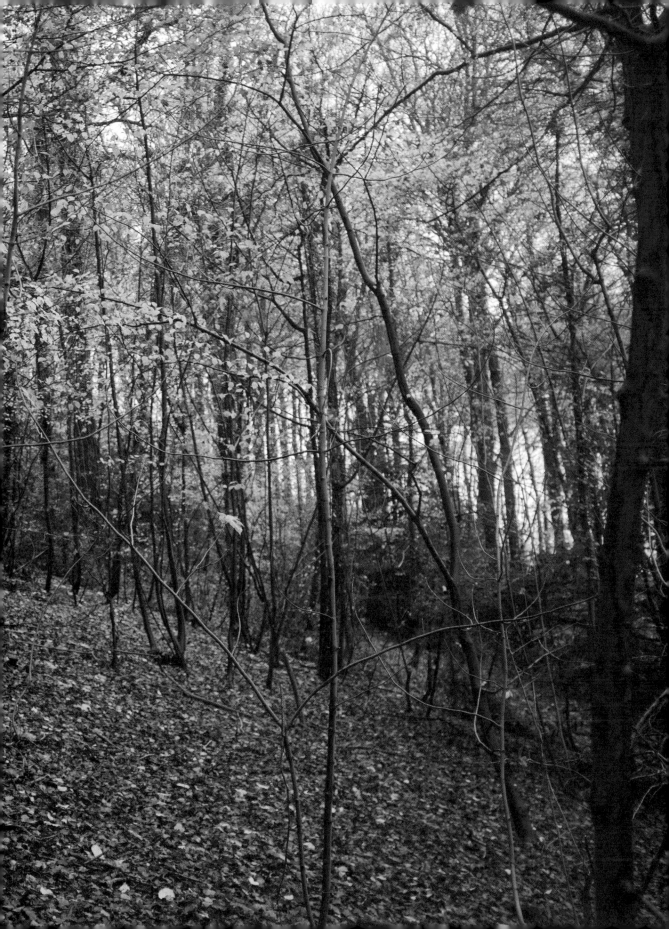

Forest bathing in different seasons

Spring

- Notice the new growth on the trees, plants and flowers
- Listen to birdsong
- Enjoy the warmth of the sun
- Smell fresh spring air and notice which aromas you can pick out
- Notice the increased animal activity
- Observe newly emerging blooms (bluebells and snowdrops are big hits!)

Summer

- Smell the flowers blossoming
- Feel the rain on your skin
- Spend longer in the forest (if you can, three hours is great!)
- Notice different shades of green
- Feel the difference between the sun and the shade
- Relax in the coolness of the forest on a hot day

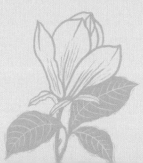
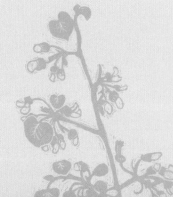

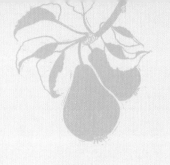

Autumn

- Smell the fallen leaves
- Watch the leaves changing colours
- Create nature art out of fallen leaves, conkers and acorns
- Feel the wind on your skin
- Crunch fallen leaves in your hands and listen to the sound they make
- Smell the soil and leaf litter

Winter

- Feel the cool air on your skin
- Trace bare tree branches with your eyes
- Listen to the sound of the frozen soil underneath your feet as you walk
- Watch the frost melt in the morning
- Watch the dew drops on the trees
- Enjoy the magic of freshly fallen snow in a forest

Endnotes

1 Li Q., Morimoto K., Nakadai A., Inagaki H., Katsumata M., Shimizu T., Hirata Y., Hirata K., Suzuki H., Miyazaki Y., Kagawa T., Koyama Y., Ohira T., Takayama N., Krensky A.M., Kawada T., 'Forest bathing enhances human natural killer activity and expression of anti-cancer proteins', *International Journal of Immunopathology and Pharmacology*, 2007 Apr-Jun, 20(2 Suppl 2):3-8, doi: 10.1177/03946320070200S202, PMID: 17903349.

2 Mathew P. White, Ian Alcock, Benedict W. Wheeler, Michael Depledge, 'Would You Be Happier Living in a Greener Urban Area? A Fixed-Effects Analysis of Panel Data', *Psychological Science* 24(6), April 2013, doi:10.1177/095679761246465, PubMed.

3 Jamie Broadley, Jenn Barnett, Karl Simons OBE, Charles Alberts, Dr Richard Heron, Steve Bird, Sarah Restall, Dr Stephanie Fitzgerald, Simon Blake OBE, Rob Stephenson, Sean Maywood, Simon Jay, Jack Green Oly, Laura Dallas, Harry Corin, Wendy Robinson, Alice Hendy, Francis Goss, Louise Aston, Ryan Briggs, Richard Jackson, Daniella Brackpool, Julie Robinson, Andy Holmes, Zoe Eccleston, Sandy-Lee Connolly, Gethin Nadin, Paul Dockerty, Arti Kashyap-Aynsley, Hayley Farrell, Beth Samson, Jonathan Gawthrop, Nick Davison, Jamie Douglas, Ryan Hopkins, Jake Sanders, *The Workplace Health Report 2023*, Champion Health, 2023. This study collected data between January and October 2022 from 4,170 employees across the globe. This consisted of over 1,000,000 data points covering all areas of wellbeing.

4 Zhang D., Lee E.K.P., Mak E.C.W., Ho C.Y., Wong S.Y.S., 'Mindfulness-based interventions: an overall review', *British Medical Bulletin*, June 2021, 138(1), pp. 41–57, https://doi.org/10.1093/bmb/ldab005.

5 Clarke, F.J., Kotera, Y., McEwan, K., 'A Qualitative Study Comparing Mindfulness and Shinrin-Yoku (Forest Bathing): Practitioners' Perspectives', *Sustainability*, June 2021, 13:6761, https://doi.org/10.3390/su13126761.

6 Easter, M., *The Comfort Crisis: Embrace Discomfort To Reclaim Your Wild, Happy, Healthy Self*, Rodale Books, 2021.

7 Hopman, R.J., 'Measuring Cognition in Nature: An Exploratory Study Using Electroencephalograpgy: A thesis submitted to the faculty of The University of Utah in partial fulfilment of the requirements for the degree of Master of Science', Department of Psychology, The University of Utah, August 2016.

8 Hunter M.R., Gillespie B.W., Chen SY.-P., 'Urban Nature Experiences Reduce Stress in the Context of Daily Life Based on Salivary Biomarkers', *Frontiers in Psychology*, 2019, 10:722, doi: 10.3389/fpsyg.2019.00722.

9 Cited in Easter, M., 'The '20-5-3' Rule Prescribes How Much Time to Spend Outside', *Men's Health*, 4 June, 2021, www.menshealth.com/fitness/a36547849/how-much-time-should-i-spend-outside/.

10 Liisa Tyrväinen, Ann Ojala, Kalevi Korpela, Timo Lanki, Yuko Tsunetsugu, Takahide Kagawa, 'The influence of urban green environments on stress relief

measures: A field experiment', *Journal of Environmental Psychology*, Volume 38, 2014, pages 1-9, ISSN 0272-4944, https://doi.org/10.1016/j.jenvp.2013.12.005.

[11] Li, Q., 'Effect of forest bathing trips on human immune function', *Environmental Health and Preventative Medicine* 15, 9–17, 2010, https://doi.org/10.1007/s12199-008-0068-3.

[12] Kirsten McEwan, David Giles, Fiona J. Clarke, Yasu Kotera, Gary Evans, Olga Terebenina, Lina Minou, Claire Teeling, Jaskaran Basran, Wendy Wood, et al., 'A Pragmatic Controlled Trial of Forest Bathing Compared with Compassionate Mind Training in the UK: Impacts on Self-Reported Wellbeing and Heart Rate Variability', *Sustainability* 13, no. 3: 1380, 2021, https://doi.org/10.3390/su13031380.

[13] Clifford, M.A., *Your Guide to Forest Bathing (Expanded Edition): Experience the Healing Power of Nature*, Red Wheel/Weiser, 2021.

[14] Li Q., Kobayashi M., Wakayama Y., Inagaki H., Katsumata M., Hirata Y., Hirata K., Shimizu T., Kawada T., Park B.J., Ohira T., Kagawa T., Miyazaki Y., 'Effect of phytoncide from trees on human natural killer cell function', *International Journal of Immunopathology and Pharmacology*, 2009, 22(4):951–9, https://journals.sagepub.com/doi/10.1177/039463200902200410.

[15] Simard S., Perry D., Jones M., et al., 'Net transfer of carbon between ectomycorrhizal tree species in the field', *Nature* 388, 579–582, 1997, https://doi.org/10.1038/41557.

[16] George MacKerron, Susana Mourato, 'Happiness is greater in natural environments', *Global Environmental Change*, 23 (5), pp. 992-1000, 2013, ISSN 0959-3780.

[17] Liu Kexiu, Mohamed Elsadek, Binyi Liu, Eijiro Fujii, 'Foliage colors improve relaxation and emotional status of university students from different countries', *Heliyon*, Volume 7, Issue 1, 2021, e06131, ISSN 2405-8440, https://doi.org/10.1016/j.heliyon.2021.e06131; University of Sussex and G.F. Smith's 'World's Favourite Colour' survey into 26,596 people from more than 100 countries, 2019.

[18] R.P. Taylor, 'Reduction of Physiological Stress Using Fractal Art and Architecture', Massachusetts Institute of Technology, *Leonardo* 39 (3): 245–251, https://doi.org/10.1162/leon.2006.39.3.245, 2006.

[19] Hagerhall C.M., Laike T., Taylor R.P., Küller M., Küller R., Martin T.P., 'Investigations of human EEG response to viewing fractal patterns', *Perception*, 37(10):1488-94, 2008, doi: 10.1068/p5918. PMID: 19065853.

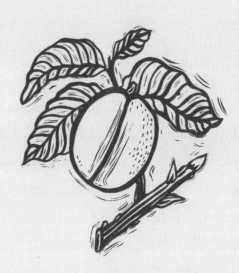

[20] Jo, H., Song, C., Miyazaki, Y. 'Physiological Benefits of Viewing Nature: A Systematic Review of Indoor Experiments', *International Journal of Environmental Research and Public Health*, 16(23):4739, 2019, https://doi.org/10.3390/ijerph16234739.

[21] Blum W.E.H,. Zechmeister-Boltenstern S., Keiblinger K.M., 'Does Soil Contribute to the Human Gut Microbiome?', *Microorganisms*, 2019 Aug 23;7(9):287, doi: 10.3390/microorganisms7090287, PMID: 31450753; PMCID: PMC6780873.

[22] Katarzyna Socała, Urszula Doboszewska, Aleksandra Szopa, Anna Serefko, Marcin Włodarczyk, Anna Zielińska, Ewa Poleszak, Jakub Fichna, Piotr Wlaź, 'The role of microbiota-gut-brain axis in neuropsychiatric and neurological disorders', *Pharmacological Research*, Volume 172, 2021, 105840, ISSN 1043-6618, https://doi.org/10.1016/j.phrs.2021.105840.

[23] Shukla S.D., Budden K.F., Neal R., Hansbro P.M., 'Microbiome effects on immunity, health and disease in the lung', *Clinical & Translational Immunology*, 6: e133, 2017, https://doi.org/10.1038/cti.2017.6.

[24] Oschman J.L., Chevalier G., Brown R., 'The effects of grounding (earthing) on inflammation, the immune response, wound healing, and prevention and treatment of chronic inflammatory and autoimmune diseases', *Journal of Inflammation Research*, 2015 Mar 24;8:83-96, doi: 10.2147/JIR.S69656, PMID: 25848315; PMCID: PMC4378297.

[25] Chevalier, G., 'The effect of grounding the human body on mood', *Psychological Reports*, 2015 Apr;116(2):534-42, doi: 10.2466/06.PR0.116k21w5, Epub 2015 Mar 6, PMID: 25748085.

[26] Ghaly M., Teplitz D., 'The biological effects of grounding the human body during sleep, as measured by cortisol levels and subjective reporting of sleep, pain and stress', *Journal of Alternative and Complementary Medicine*, 2004 10(5):767-776; Chevalier G., Mori K., Oschman J., 'The effect of Earthing (grounding) on human physiology', *European Biology and Bioelectromagnetics* Jan 31, 2006; 600-621.

[27] Ibid, 24.

[28] Barrable, A., Booth, D., Adams, D., Beauchamp, B., 'Enhancing Nature Connection and Positive Affect in Children through Mindful Engagement with Natural Environments', *International Journal of Environmental Research and Public Health*, 2021, 18(9):4785, https://doi.org/10.3390/ijerph18094785.

[29] Information from the article 'Children & Nature Programme: the importance of integrating time spent in nature at school' by Martin Gilchrist for Natural England, 16 May 2023, https://naturalengland.blog.gov.uk/2023/05/16/.

[30] Stephen Kaplan, 'The restorative benefits of nature: Toward an integrative framework', *Journal of Environmental Psychology*, Volume 15, Issue 3, 1995, pp. 169-182, ISSN 0272-4944, https://doi.org/10.1016/0272-4944(95)90001-2.

[31] Nalini M. Nadkarni, Patricia H. Hasbach, Tierney Thys, Emily Gaines Crockett, Lance Schnacker, 'Impacts of nature imagery on people in severely nature-deprived environments',

Frontiers in Ecology and the Environment, 2017, https://doi.org/10.1002/fee.1518.

[32] Armitage C.J., 'Can the theory of planned behavior predict the maintenance of physical activity?', *Health Psychology*, May 2005, 24(3):235-45, doi: 10.1037/0278-6133.24.3.235.

[33] Lardone A., Liparoti M., Sorrentino P., Rucco R., Jacini F., Polverino A., Minino R., Pesoli M., Baselice F., Sorriso A., Ferraioli G., Sorrentino G., Mandolesi L., 'Mindfulness Meditation Is Related to Long-Lasting Changes in Hippocampal Functional Topology during Resting State: A Magnetoencephalography Study', *Neural Plasticity*, 2018 Dec 18;2018:5340717, doi: 10.1155/2018/5340717, PMID: 30662457; PMCID: PMC6312586.

[34] World Wildlife Fund, *Living Planet Report 2024*, https://livingplanet.panda.org/en-US/.

[35] Hannah Ritchie, 'The world has lost one-third of its forest, but an end of deforestation is possible', published online at OurWorldinData.org, 2021. Retrieved from: www.ourworldindata.org/world-lost-one-third-forests, 9 December 2024.

[36] FAO and UNEP, *The State of the World's Forests 2020: Forests, biodiversity and people*, Rome, https://doi.org/10.4060/ca8642en.

[37] Data taken from the article 'State of Nature' by Dr Pete Brotherton for Natural England, 29 September 2023, http://naturalengland.blog.gov.uk/2023/09/29/.

[38] Burns F., Mordue S., al Fulaij N., Boersch-Supan P.H., Boswell J., Boyd R.J., Bradfer-Lawrence T., de Ornellas P., de Palma A., de Zylva P., Dennis E.B., Foster S., Gilbert G., Halliwell L., Hawkins K., Haysom K.A., Holland M.M., Hughes J., Jackson A.C., Mancini F., Mathews F., McQuatters-Gollop A., Noble D.G., O'Brien D., Pescott O.L., Purvis A., Simkin J., Smith A., Stanbury A.J., Villemot J., Walker K.J., Walton P., Webb T.J., Williams J., Wilson R., Gregory R.D., *State of Nature 2023*, State of Nature Partnership, available at: www.stateofnature.org.uk.

[39] Information from the press release 'In the ten worst-hit countries, increasing floods and drought have forced people to flee 8 million times last year – over twice that of a decade ago', published on Oxfam.org, 20 June 2024.

[40] Caroline M.L. Mackay, Michael T. Schmitt, 'Do people who feel connected to nature do more to protect it? A meta-analysis', *Journal of Environmental Psychology*, Volume 65, 2019, 101323, ISSN 0272-4944, https://doi.org/10.1016/j.jenvp.2019.101323.

[41] Most of these systemic reviews can be found in the *Journal of Happiness Studies*.

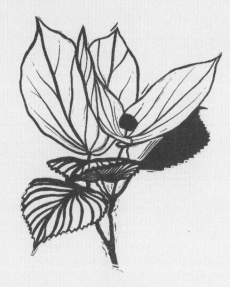

About the authors

Olga Terebenina

Olga Terebenina is a peer-reviewed nature author and researcher, co-founder of The Forest Bathing Institute, World Economic Forum Top Innovator, one of the Top 100 Global Women Entrepreneurs 2024 in *Global Woman Magazine*, and an environmental activist.

From early childhood, Olga was interested in nature and ways we can protect and enhance natural environments. When faced with health problems in her late teens, she turned to nature. She found that spending time in nature was not only an effective solution for her health problems, but that these findings were backed by research and could, in turn, inspire a movement to help protect habitats for current and future generations.

In 2018, together with her husband Gary Evans, Olga set up The Forest Bathing Institute (TFBI), a world leader in research, events and training on nature's health and wellbeing benefits.

TFBI has established links with around 100 universities worldwide, including Harvard University, UCL, King's College, London, and Nippon Medical School in Tokyo, Japan, all with numerous research programmes underway. The Institute also works to raise awareness of the effectiveness of nature therapy. It works closely with local and central governments, the NHS in the UK, charities and key policymakers to make Forest Bathing+ (a slow, mindful walk in the woodland, where you are guided through a series of sensory experiences proven to reduce stress and anxiety) available to as many people who can benefit as possible.

Olga has been featured on *People Fixing the World* (BBC Sounds), *Stories of Us* (BBC Two), *The Wellbeing Lab with Will Young* (Acast), and the MUD\WTR *Trends with Benefits* podcast. Olga plans to continue spreading the word about the benefits of spending time in nature and ecological protection to communities while working with the media, governments and universities worldwide.

Gary Evans

Gary Evans, director and co-founder of The Forest Bathing Institute, is a peer-reviewed author and researcher on the health benefits of forest bathing.

Gary pioneered Forest Bathing+ alongside his wife Olga. Together, they have led hundreds of forest bathing sessions for the general public, health care professionals, NHS staff, Defra, Natural England, Forestry England, county councils, universities and world experts in nature therapy.

Gary regularly consults with governments, universities, healthcare providers, wildlife charities and landowners. He is regularly quoted in the national and international press and featured in countless publications, including *The Guardian* and *The Telegraph*. His media appearances include BBC TV, BBC Earth and BBC Radio.

Gary's love of nature started at a young age, something he credits to his father. He has an inquisitive mind and likes to understand things, rather than just accepting how things appear to be. When Gary looks at forests, birds and animals, he is amazed and moved by the beauty he sees and feels. This worldview formed the foundation for The Forest Bathing Institute. He always wondered if there were health benefits to spending time in forests and could not understand why these benefits were not widely understood or studied extensively. After all, understanding our connection to nature is the most natural thing. The discovery of forest bathing joined big dots, and Gary's research began.

Gary's determination to confirm that the Japanese scientific studies behind forest bathing can be applied in England led to his being credited as a researcher for the University of Derby. He now regularly consults with universities across the world with the aim of helping as many people as possible, reminding them of the priceless wonders that nature has to offer all of us, and beseeching them from the bottom of his heart to help save what little is left, for themselves and for future generations.

If you are reading this, please meditate (ideally under a tree) on humans and your role as caretakers of the environment.

To find out more about The Forest Bathing Institute and the latest research and developments in forest bathing, please see our website: **www.tfb.institute**.

About the photographer and illustrator

Dominick Tyler

Dominick's photography career started in student media while he was studying Philosophy at UCL and quickly led to freelance work for national newspapers, in the years that followed he built up a long list of editorial, commercial and NGO clients.

His long-term project *The Edge of Two Worlds*, documenting the changing lives of a community of Innu in northern Canada, won the Marty Forscher Fellowship Award for Humanistic Photography in 2005, and second place in *The Observer* Hodge award in 2004. This work was published internationally and exhibited in the Leica galleries in Frankfurt and Solms, and in the Proud Gallery in London.

In 2007 Dominick collaborated with writer Kate Rew on the best-selling book *Wild Swim*, which was credited with launching an outdoor swimming revival. Dominick wrote and photographed *Uncommon Ground*, which was published by Guardian Faber in 2015 to wide acclaim – described by George Monbiot as '…an astonishing book of heart-wrenching beauty, which will re-ignite your enchantment with the natural world.'

Rosanna Morris

Rosanna Morris has worked in the realm of print for well over ten years. She first got excited about relief print at eighteen during her foundation diploma at the Bristol School of Art. During the course she took a trip to Paris where she encountered inspiring large-scale street art around the city. Once home she wanted to make her drawings big and began carving huge life size woodcuts of British farming and pasted them on abandoned walls around the city. She went on to study Illustration at Camberwell College of Arts, where she developed her own unique style, evoking the traditional feel of British Wood Engravings within the aesthetic of contemporary illustration.

Acknowledgements

We are very grateful to Professor Sara Warber and Dr Katherine Irvine for believing in our work in 2016 when forest bathing research in Europe and North America was still in its infancy.

We will be forever grateful to Professor Qing Li for inspiring us to explore forest bathing, for his groundbreaking research into its benefits, and for his friendship and support.

We are also thankful to Professor Miles Richardson and Associate Professor Kirsten McEwan at the University of Derby, without whom some of our initial research projects would not have been possible, as well as Amos Clifford, the founder of ANFT, for his inspiring work in forest therapy.

We are also grateful to everyone in government departments and the NHS who understood the value of nature-based therapies and supported us. A special mention to Surrey County Council and Jane Soothill. We want to thank the charities and land owners we have worked with, including the Wildlife Trusts, National Trust, the RSPB, Forestry England, Woodland Trust, Catalyst Mental Health, Amber and others, for their support and for allowing us to use their land to run forest bathing sessions and to conduct our research.

We are very grateful to our forest bathing event participants and forest bathing guide students, who, thanks to their feedback, helped us develop our sessions to maximize the therapeutic benefits of the practice.

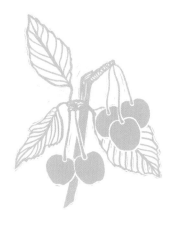

A huge thanks to the whole TFBI team; your help and support throughout the years means more than words can convey. We appreciate you believing in our work, helping to build our organization and inspiring others to connect with nature.

Many thanks to our Ayurveda and Vedic studies teacher, Acharya Shunya, and to Aparna Amy Lewis for deepening our understanding of nature, both external and our own.

Big thanks to our yoga teacher Yogi Manish Singh, and to Paramahansa Yogananda and Self-Realization Fellowship whose yogic teachings harnessed and inspired our mindfulness-based approach in forest bathing.

We are very grateful to our editor Sophie Lazar, Katerina Menhennet, and the Quarto Group team for their all their hard work, patience and care in creating this book.

Thousands of people have supported our journey, a heartfelt thanks to everyone we have not mentioned.

We are also grateful to our family for their unceasing support and patience in watching us grow our organization.

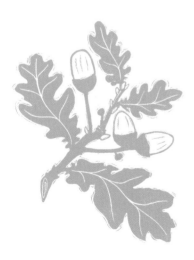

Further reading

Kabat-Zinn, Jon. *Full Catastrophe Living: How to cope with stress, pain and illness using mindfulness meditation* (Revised edition), Piatkus, 2013.

Leon, Natalie. *The Japanese Art of Living Seasonally: An Invitation to Celebrate Every Day*, Watkins Publishing, 2024.

Li, Dr Qing. *Into the Forest: How Trees Can Help You Find Health and Happiness*, Penguin Books UK, 2019.

Li, Dr Qing. *Shinrin-Yoku: The Art and Science of Forest Bathing*, Penguin Books UK, 2018.

Ober, Clinton; Sinatra, Stephen T.; Zucker, Martin; Oschman, James L., *Earthing: The most important health discovery ever!* (Second edition), Basic Health Publications, Inc, 2014.

Richardson Miles. *Reconnection: Fixing our Broken Relationship with Nature*, Pelagic Publishing, 2023.

Simard, Suzanne. *Finding the Mother Tree: Uncovering the Wisdom and Intelligence of the Forest*, Penguin Books UK, 2022.

Williams, Florence. *The Nature Fix: Why Nature Makes Us Happier, Healthier, and More Creative*, W. W. Norton & Company, 2017.

Wohlleben, Peter. *The Hidden Life of Trees: What They Feel, How They Communicate*, William Collins, 2017.

Index